Environmental Monitoring for Cleanrooms and Controlled Environments

DRUGS AND THE PHARMACEUTICAL SCIENCES

A Series of Textbooks and Monographs

Executive Editor

James Swarbrick

PharmaceuTech, Inc.
Pinehurst, North Carolina

Advisory Board

Larry L. Augsburger
University of Maryland
Baltimore, Maryland

Harry G. Brittain
Center for Pharmaceutical Physics
Milford, New Jersey

Jennifer B. Dressman
Johann Wolfgang Goethe University
Frankfurt, Germany

Anthony J. Hickey
University of North Carolina School of
Pharmacy
Chapel Hill, North Carolina

Jeffrey A. Hughes
University of Florida College of
Pharmacy
Gainesville, Florida

Ajaz Hussain
Sandoz
Princeton, New Jersey

Trevor M. Jones
The Association of the
British Pharmaceutical Industry
London, United Kingdom

Stephen G. Schulman
University of Florida
Gainesville, Florida

Vincent H. L. Lee
University of Southern California
Los Angeles, California

Elizabeth M. Topp
University of Kansas School of
Pharmacy
Lawrence, Kansas

Jerome P. Skelly
Alexandria, Virginia

Peter York
University of Bradford School of
Pharmacy
Bradford, United Kingdom

Geoffrey T. Tucker
University of Sheffield
Royal Hallamshire Hospital
Sheffield, United Kingdom

Environmental Monitoring for Cleanrooms and Controlled Environments

edited by

Anne Marie Dixon

Cleanroom Management Associates, Inc.
Carson City, Nevada, U.S.A.

informa

healthcare

New York   London

Foreword

As with many aspects of scientific endeavor, the passage of time often provides deeper knowledge, greater clarity, and understanding. Take for example the discovery of microbes, or germs, as the causative agent for infection. Louis Pasteur demonstrated that the fermentation process was caused by the growth of microorganisms and that the growth of microorganisms in nutrient broths was not a result of spontaneous generation. With his experiments, he managed to convince most of Europe that the germ theory of disease, also called the pathogenic theory of medicine as the cause of many infectious diseases, was true. This clearer understanding of the cause of disease opened new doors for innovation in hygienic practices and the development of antibiotics. The passage of time, to some extent, has done this for the subject of environmental monitoring.

In the past two decades, technological advances have taken active air sampling from a cumbersome activity with relatively primitive equipment in a cleanroom environment to a simple process with self-contained, easily sanitized sampling devices. Particle monitoring that required operators to remain stationary during a filling process and document counts manually have been replaced with sophisticated remote-sensing devices that can record, analyze, and maintain data with little to no human intervention. The understanding of how, where, when, and why to sample and analyze data has also improved.

Conversely, our advanced communication technology has resulted in the promulgation of reams of available information. Attempting to remain current with this potential deluge has presented challenges to those responsible for environmental monitoring programs. Regulatory guidance documents have become more numerous and, although efforts at harmonization continue, are not consistent. As a result, there is more information available to digest, but there is not a concomitant, automatic level of understanding to go with it.

The lack of a clear understanding of the purpose of an environmental monitoring program and its relationship to the release of a sterile pharmaceutical product can end up as a very costly error and waste of good product, or, more seriously, pose a potential health risk to the patient. Within the framework of risk management, environmental monitoring is considered a very important mitigation measure for manufacturers of sterile products. Thus, having a firm foundational understanding of this important program is essential to an overall sterility assurance program.

This guide is an invaluable resource for helping to provide the clarity of understanding of key aspects of environmental monitoring. There is a significant body of available information related to this topic. This book focuses on presenting clear, simple, practical information in an easy-to-read format. The first section of the book encompasses the basics of how particles and microbes behave in a cleanroom. Understanding this behavior is vital in establishing a meaningful and effective environmental monitoring program. Helping wend the way through the expanding guidance documents, it provides clear information on the new International Standards Organization standards and their application as another key building block for the environmental monitoring program. Chapters on particle, viable air, and surface monitoring provide considerations for equipment selection, their operation, maintenance, data generation, and, most importantly, data analysis and management. Monitoring of water and related endotoxin are also included.

Regulatory agencies around the globe have expectations for any product purported to be sterile. The sterility testing that is required is one of the most important for the release of product, and while the sterility test has its limitations, false positives can result in the unnecessary rejection of product; hence, it is critical to understand the essential requirements for this test. Associated with this are the expectations for final drug products produced utilizing aseptic processing. Aseptic processing simulations, or media fills, though seemingly simple procedures, require clear understanding in order to construct and conduct ones that will address all the requirements to provide the data that supports the ongoing acceptability of the process. In essence, aseptic processing and its associated controls replace terminal sterilization of products. In this book, the reader will find chapters that address each of these in clear and concise terms.

It has been my privilege to work with Anne Marie Dixon for nearly two decades. Her depth of knowledge of environmental monitoring, as well as the broader topic of cleanroom standards, is nothing short of inspirational. With this book, she has brought together a group of experts who have created a deep, practical, and easily understandable reservoir of information that should provide the user with the knowledge needed to utilize environmental monitoring in the manner it was intended—as an ongoing indicator of environmental and process control. This book provides that deeper knowledge, greater clarity, and understanding of the subject.

Nanette Londeree
Formerly of Bayer,
Pharmaceutical Division,
Biological Products,
Berkeley, California, U.S.A.

Preface

Contamination, which causes product defects, is a measurable process variable. It is defined today as any material, substance, or energy that adversely affects a product or process. The science of contamination control is a multidisciplinary technology drawing on chemistry, physics, material science, microbiology, and other fields. One of the critical technologies in this field is environmental monitoring.

Environmental monitoring is a tool that provides meaningful information on the quality of a process, processing environment, and final product. An adequate program will aid the user of cleanrooms and controlled environments to identify and eliminate potential sources of contamination. Parts 211 and 600 of Title 21 of the Code of Federal Regulations include general requirements for environmental control of pharmaceutical and biological processes. However, bulk manufacturing and medical device industries must also monitor their processes and environments.

Many guidance documents are often open to interpretation. In addition, there are scattered industry standards, technical reports, International Standards Organization standards, and other documents that offer some assistance.

This book was developed to assist the user by providing information on the entire subject of environmental monitoring and the interpretation of this data as a tool in the field of contamination control. An environmental monitoring program generally includes the monitoring of air (both viable and nonviable), surfaces, water, alert and action levels, trending, and procedures for responding to excursions. This book also includes information on certification/requalification and the new International Standards Organization standards. Chapter 1 presents background information on how aerosols perform in cleanrooms or controlled environments.

Written procedures exist in today's manufacturing facilities, addressing such areas as frequency of sampling, location of sample, time of sampling, conditions, duration, sample size, and techniques. The interpretation of the results is key in controlling contamination. Several chapters address the data presentation, trending, and investigations and how they can provide a valuable tool in reducing risk to product, process, and patient.

Cleanrooms and controlled environments do not operate themselves. They must be maintained, supported, controlled, and carefully monitored. The cleanroom is a tool that is used to eliminate variables by providing a stable and safe background environment for our products. An environmental monitoring program can become a valuable tool to assist both quality and manufacturing departments in reducing the risk to product and processes.

Anne Marie Dixon

Contents

Contributors

David Brande   NNE-US, Inc., Clayton, North Carolina, U.S.A.

Anne Marie Dixon   Cleanroom Management Associates, Inc., Carson City, Nevada, U.S.A.

David S. Ensor   Center for Aerosol Technology, RTI International, Research Triangle Park, North Carolina, U.S.A.

Karin K. Foarde   Microbial and Molecular Biology, RTI International, Research Triangle Park, North Carolina, U.S.A.

Bengt Ljungqvist   Building Services Engineering, KTH, Stockholm, Sweden

Richard A. Matthews   Filtration Technology, Inc., Greensboro, North Carolina, U.S.A.

Karen Zink McCullough   Whitehouse Station, New Jersey, U.S.A.

Berit Reinmüller   Building Services Engineering, KTH, Stockholm, Sweden

Scott Sutton   Vectech Pharmaceutical Consultants, Farmington Hills, Michigan, U.S.A.

Audra Zakzeski   Carson City, Nevada, U.S.A.

1 The Behavior of Particles in Cleanrooms

David S. Ensor and Karin K. Foarde

1   The Behavior of Particles in Cleanrooms

David S. Ensor
Center for Aerosol Technology, RTI International, Research Triangle Park, North Carolina, U.S.A.

Karin K. Foarde
Microbial and Molecular Biology, RTI International, Research Triangle Park, North Carolina, U.S.A.

INTRODUCTION

Background

The specification and design of cleanroom environmental monitoring programs should consider behavior of particles with respect to sources, transport, and fate. Although a cleanroom represents a controlled environment with unidirectional flow and highly filtered air, the location of particle sources within the room, equipment, and personnel may influence the transport of particles and may affect critical processing locations.

Monitoring programs to quantify particle concentration need to recognize potential particle size-dependent sampling and measurement biases. Gravitational settling rates and particle inertia depend on the particle diameter, shape, and specific gravity. Sedimentation or gravitational settling may affect the location and concentration of particles in the cleanroom. Sampling particles may have particle size-dependent errors from entry of particles from the cleanroom air to sampling inlets from inertia. Settling of particles in sampling tubing and inertial deposition on tubing bends in the sampler may also cause particle size-dependent biases of the sample.

Cleanroom Airflow

Cleanrooms may be configured in many different ways depending on the intended purpose. The performance of the cleanroom depends on the type of airflow design (turbulent or unidirectional flow), location of air inlets and return, and size and location of processing equipment. The diagram of a unidirectional flow cleanroom operation in Figure 1A illustrates a simple layout with ceiling filters and side returns. Clean air from the inlet filters displaces and removes contaminating particles from the work area. Sources of particles in the cleanroom include potential pathways through leaks around the filters, direct penetration through the filters, the processes, reentrainment from surfaces, and shedding from operators.

ISO 14644-4 (1) contains minimum requirements for design and construction. Airborne cleanliness standards and monitoring are covered by ISO 14644-1 and -2 (2,3). Biocontamination requirements are in ISO 14698-1 and -2 (4,5). A cleanroom may be evaluated under three possible conditions or states: as-built, at-rest, and operational. The as-built state describes a functioning cleanroom without process equipment. The at-rest state includes process equipment without activity. The operational state describes the situation of full production activity. Particles in a

(A)

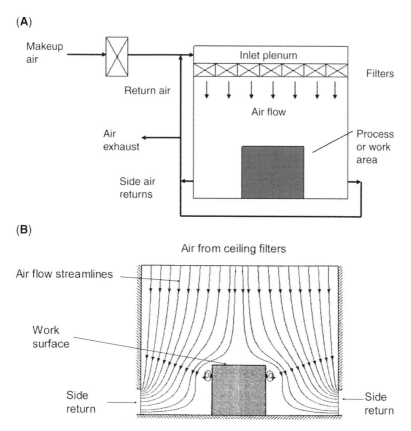

(B)

FIGURE 1 (**A**) Diagram of a unidirectional flow cleanroom illustrating relative location of inlets, returns, and airflow. Air-conditioning, fans, and dampers have not been shown for clarity. (**B**) Computation of cleanroom airflow streamlines. Formation of an eddy at the corner of the work area.

working cleanroom may follow complex paths in the presence of operating equipment and personnel.

Some insights can be gained from airflow-modeling results. An example of airflow modeling developed by Yamamoto et al. (6,7) is shown in Figure 1B. The model used a two-dimensional Navier–Stokes solution to the equations of flow. Particles generally follow the streamlines of airflow. However, sufficiently large particles may settle by gravity or have sufficient mass or inertia to deviate from the airflow when the air changes direction. In Figure 1B, the flow streamlines are shown for the case of a full-filtered ceiling with wall side returns. The air is shown flowing around an obstacle such as a solid table or process equipment. At the edges of the obstacle in this particular example, recirculation zones form. Recirculation of air may cause transport of particles from the floor to the top of the work surface. Although a cleanroom maybe designed to provide unidirectional airflow, the presence of and operation of processing equipment and people in a working facility can change the character of the airflow. Fitzner (8) demonstrated the complexity of airflow in a cleanroom with smoke-tracer experiments. For example, airflow around obstacles was demonstrated to cause a wake with eddies and mixing. Also people in the cleanroom create disturbances or wakes associated with their movement.

Cleanroom Monitoring
Cleanroom particle cleanliness monitoring uses optical particle counters to measure the number of particles larger than a specific particle size (e.g., 0.5 μm) per cubic meter of air as the metric. This count includes all particles of this specific size range regardless of the source and properties. Cleanroom monitoring specifically for microorganisms requires specialized sampling equipment to deposit the particles on a growth media and posttreatment to quantify colonies. Microorganisms are a special case of particles in a cleanroom. When microorganisms are airborne, they are often referred to as bioaerosols. Although the definition of bioaerosols is quite broad and covers many diverse organisms and components of those organisms, this discussion will be limited to bacteria and fungi. Bioaerosols differ in many ways from the common picture of particles as smooth, spherical, and solid. They are alive and can reproduce, are frequently nonspherical, and have a number of other nonideal physical characteristics and properties.

PHYSICAL PROPERTIES OF PARTICLES

Size and Shape
Particle size has the most significant effect on particle behavior. Properties affected by size include settling rate, adhesion, mobility, light scattering from the particle, and electrical charging. Liquids will form spherical particles by the effect of surface tension. However, solid particles are rarely perfect spheres. Often the shape of the particles may affect physical and chemical properties as well because very irregular or porous particles will have increased surface areas. Therefore, the particle density may be quite different from the density of the bulk materials.

    The reported diameter is often an equivalent diameter, which depends on the measurement method. An equivalent diameter is the diameter of the sphere that would have the same value of a particular physical property as that of the irregular particle. Sizing instruments may use properties of the particle such as mass, optical light scattering, and electrical charge to deduce a size. After collection of the particles on a suitable substrate, microscopic methods may be used to determine an image or a physical diameter.

Composition
Composition affects the physical and chemical/biological properties of the particles. Composition depends on the source of the particles and how they are generated and the distance from the source. Transport often involves dilution of the particles and losses to surfaces. The composition of the particles may be related to potential detrimental effects of the particle. One of the objectives of a monitoring program is to identify the type and sources of particles.

Concentration
Typically when monitoring airborne particles, the concentration of the particles per volume of gas is critical. The measurement depends on measuring both the number of particles and the volume of gas.

Particle Size Distributions

Airborne particles are rarely found as a single-particle size. Even a group of one type of microorganism will exhibit a distribution in size because of natural variability. Sometimes, organisms or particles may be clumped creating larger particles from the formation process or Brownian coagulation while airborne. By necessity, the results need to be treated statistically. In the cumulative format, the particle size distribution is plotted as the numbers of particles "larger than or equal to" a specific diameter or the cumulative numbers of particle "smaller than or equal to" a specific diameter. The "larger than or equal to" cumulative curves are used in the cleanroom industry to define cleanliness standards (2). This convention was likely motivated by limitations in instrumentation. It is a reasonable assumption that particles larger than a specific diameter will be detected by an optical particle counter. The particles smaller than a specific lower limit cannot be detected because of resolution limitations of the instrument. Often particle size distributions are fitted with mathematical models to better understand behavior. The straight line used in cleanroom standards in logarithmic coordinates is an example of a power law distribution:

$$N(d_p) = d_p^{-n} \tag{1}$$

where $N(d_p)$ is the cumulative number distribution as a function of particle diameter, d_p the particle diameter, and n a statistically determined slope of the size distribution.

Size distributions are characterized with moments, mean, mode, and standard deviations. Often logarithmic distributions are used to characterize the observed sizes. For more information, please refer to Ensor (9) and Hinds (10). For scientific work, often the size increment is normalized with a log increment to cause the area under the curve in log–log plot to relate to a parameter of interest.

Inert Particle Formation

The formation processes determine both the composition and the size. Mechanical processes such as abrasion, crushing, and grinding are normally responsible for particles larger than 1 μm. These larger particles may be introduced into the air immediately upon formation or introduced by resuspension from the floor or other surfaces. Particles smaller than 1 μm normally are formed by gas-phase chemical reactions or the condensation of vapor. Particles may be formed from spray droplets as dissolved solids evaporate leaving residue; the size of the particle depends on the concentration of the material in the liquid.

Biological Particles

Bioaerosols as a group vary markedly in size or shape. Examples of shapes of common bacteria are shown in Figure 2. Microbiological textbooks traditionally give size data for microorganisms. Generally, the physical size was determined microscopically by observing the organism suspended in fluid. This, however, provides only general guidance as to the properties of a bioaerosol because the bioaerosol may not be a suspension of single particles. Rather the bioaerosol may be a suspension of microbiological particles attached to various kinds of environmental particles. These environmental particles might include dust, sputum, skin cells, etc. Therefore, the physical dimensions of microorganisms are applicable only to situations very similar to those for which the measurements were made. The aerodynamic diameters

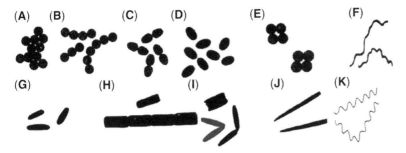

FIGURE 2 Cell shapes and arrangements for common bacterial forms. **(A)–(E)** Cocci [**(A)** staphylococci, **(B)** streptococci, **(C)** diplococci, **(D)** coccobacilli, **(E)** micrococci]; **(G)–(J)** rods [**(G)** enterobacteria, **(H)** bacilli, **(I)** coryneforms, **(J)** fusobacteria]; **(F)** and **(K)** coiled rods (spirochetes).

of bioaerosols must be directly measured. Sampling instruments are designed to collect a size range representative of the bioaerosols of interest (Table 1).

Particle properties, in addition to size and shape, may be important, although little or no data specific to microorganisms are available. For instance, the surface texture of particles may be important to their likelihood of becoming airborne. The irregular surface of a mold spore may affect its likelihood of adhering to a smooth surface. Particle density has an impact on both aerodynamics and retention on surfaces. The surrounding environment may be important. Bacteria and some fungal spores are known to change size and shape as relative humidity changes. These changes affect bioaerosol behavior.

SOURCES OF PARTICLES IN CLEANROOMS

Particle sources in the room are most likely due to local generation in the room or penetration of contaminated air from the outside through the filters. Even

TABLE 1 Representative Properties of Some Common Environmental Organisms

Organism	Type	Size and shape	Comments
Bacillus subtilis	Gram-positive bacteria	0.7–0.8 × 2–3 μm rods with an ellipsoidal spore ~0.7–0.8 × 1–1.5 μm	Spore-forming bacteria that is ubiquitous in nature
Staphylococcus epidermidis	Gram-positive bacteria	0.5–1.5 μm spheres	Vegetative bacteria which inhabits the human skin and respiratory tract
Penicillium chrysogenum	Fungus (mold)	3–4 μm × 2.8–3.8 μm, subglobose to ellipsoidal becoming globose	Found in air-conditioning systems where patients were suffering from allergic disease, food products
Cladosporium sphaerospermum	Fungus (mold)	Ellipsoidal to lemon-shaped, 3–4 × 7 μm in diameter; some ramoconidia (33 × 3–5 μm)	Found in contaminated building material, plants, soil

high-efficiency particulate air (HEPA) and ultra low penetrating air filters allow a very small fraction of particles to pass through the filter. There is always possibility of pinhole leaks in the filter, and leaks in the filter seals have not been detected and repaired. Also cleanrooms normally operate at positive pressures to prevent in leakage of contaminated air from the outside. If, for some reason, the cleanroom operates at negative pressures, leaks in the room envelope can introduce particles into the facility. The sources of particles in electronic cleanrooms were found to be evenly divided between personnel and process (11). It has also been reported that personnel contributes 35% of the contaminants (12). ISO 14644-5 (13) describes the minimum requirements for operations during manufacturing to control particles within selected limits.

Resuspension

Resuspension is, in a general sense, any process causing release of particles from a surface. The release may be caused by physical rubbing or contact with the surface, movement or flexing of the surface, vibration of the object, or the movement of gas at sufficient velocity above the surface. The detailed resuspension mechanisms are not well understood. Dynamic resuspension theory has been developed to explain detachment of inert particles from surfaces. It has been hypothesized that a population of particles have a distribution of adhesion forces with respect to the particular surface (14). In practice, when a high-velocity gas jet is used to remove particles, particle concentrations have been observed to follow an inverse time relationship t^{-1} with respect to the observed downstream concentration (15). In addition, the resuspension is dependent on the velocity of flow to exert a force on the particles and the turbulence of flow. It has been hypothesized that resuspension may be explained in terms of the airflow exerting lift on the particle in addition to simple drag to dislodge the particles from the surface (16).

   The air movement caused by walking will resuspend the particles because of the lateral airflow along the floor caused by the motion of the shoe. Although there have been limited cleanroom studies isolating this form of contamination (17), this mechanism has been shown to be important in indoor air-quality studies (18).

Nebulization

Nebulization is the formation of droplets from liquids. Whenever liquids splash or gas bubbles through a liquid, opportunities exist for generation of the particles. If droplets become airborne, the liquid will evaporate leaving an airborne solid residue. The sizes of the particles are a function of the droplet diameters and the concentration of nonvolatile residue in the liquid (11).

Thermal Processes

Particles are also formed from heating volatile material with subsequent cooling. This formation process applies to process heaters and electrical equipment (9). Although these sources are not important from a viability standpoint, the particles would contribute to the total burden of the cleanroom (11).

People

People are a significant source of particles in the cleanroom. The source particles may be found in expelled breath and shedding of particles from the skin. Masks are used to reduce the concentration of expelled breath particles. The role of cleanroom garments is to reduce the shedding of particles from people into the cleanroom. Reduction of people-generated particles, such as controlling the use of makeup, is well established. Garments are used to reduce the emissions in the room. Two parameters of interest are: particles released from the fabric and particles penetrating the fabric (19).

IEST RP-3 (20) describes the "body box method" to determine the penetration of particles through the fabric of a garment. The body box is about the size of a phone booth. Clean air is introduced into the top of the chamber, and particle sampling is conducted to measure emissions. The second method in RP-3 is the Helmke Drum test method where the garments are tumbled in a drum, and the particles released from the garment are measured with an optical particle counter. Recently, the particle size distribution of particles released from garments with the Helmke Drum test method was analyzed (21) and found to have a power law size distribution with a slope of -1 [Equation. (1)]. In addition, the method was statistically tested (22) and found to have acceptable repeatability and reproductively.

Processes in Rooms

IEST RP-26 (23) describes methods to measure particle emissions from equipment. These include a chamber and a tunnel method (24). The chamber method involves placing the device into a low leak rate chamber. Either in the chamber or connected through a duct is a blower HEPA filter combination to allow cleaning of the air and then measuring the rate of concentration build up after the flow to the filter is stopped. The duct method uses a test duct through which clean air from a fan HEPA combination flows past the device under test. The concentration of particles emitted from the device is determined by sampling the air upstream and downstream of the device. Particle emissions are reported in units of source strength, number of particle released/time, to allow application to various conditions.

Outside Air

Although cleanroom air is highly filtered, some of the particles are from the ambient outdoor environment. Viner (25) has showed that the cleanrooms tended to have a similar concentration versus time pattern as outside air with a much lower concentration under conditions of limited use. This is believed to result from the very small fraction of ambient particles penetrating the high-efficiency filters protecting the cleanroom.

Biocontaminants

Biocontaminants may become airborne in a number of ways. They may originate and become airborne outdoors and enter a building in infiltrating or make up air, be transported in from outside as a deposit and be dispersed inside, or originate and become dispersed from either inside spaces or within the ventilation system. Whatever their source, airborne biocontaminants must first become entrained in the air and then be transported. Little systematic research (specific to indoor airborne biocontaminant generation) has been conducted, but the general conditions that contribute to dispersal are known from concentration measurements and aerosol studies. The method of generation (initial dispersal) can be expected to affect the particle size and concentration.

The overall process of airborne biocontamination includes the launching step, in which biological particles are dislodged from a surface (or released by the microbiological organism) and injected into the air close to that surface; and the entrainment step, in which the now airborne biological particle is entrained in a turbulent eddy or series of eddies and carried into the mixed breathing air. Dispersed particles may settle and redeposit or become entrained in the mixed air stream and follow the air currents in the occupied space.

For fungi, the main natural method of dispersal is through the air. Many of the spore dispersal methods are quite complicated. They may be either active or passive and dry or moisture-requiring mechanisms. The minimum air speed required to remove spores from the mycelia is reported to vary from 0.4 to 2.0 m/s flow velocity. The level of turbulence and the surface velocity were not reported. A number of different spore-release mechanisms have been identified. In addition, the fungal response to falling or rising relative humidities is liberation of spores in some cases (26,27).

Some fungal spores are released as chain-like shapes, and portions of the chains could become reentrained by airflow. The rough surfaces of some other fungal spores may reduce adhesion and make them more easily resuspended. Adhesion of collected particles is significantly increased if the surface is wet with liquid such as oil or water or if a condensed interstitial water film has formed under high-humidity conditions. Extrapolating from studies of particle adhesion (28), dispersion and resuspension should be reduced by high relative humidities.

Fungal or other bioaerosols that naturally exist outdoors may enter a cleanroom duct system with incoming outdoor air or become established in a section of the duct that becomes wet or is for some reason at high humidity. If growing, fungal spores can enter the air stream. Airborne organisms that do become entrained can be transported throughout the building in the ventilation system. Bioaerosol transport through a ventilation system is similar to that of other particles having the same aerodynamic diameter. It is primarily dependent on the particle size and the system design (velocity, duct diameter, bends, etc.). A number of forces may lead to particle deposition. Large particles are likely to settle to the bottom of a duct at low-flow regions. Deposition in corners and on flow obstacles is generally caused by inertial effects (impaction). Based on theoretical analysis and experimental studies, micrometer-sized particles are probably deposited on duct walls by impaction from turbulent eddies, whereas submicrometer-sized particles are probably deposited on duct walls by Brownian diffusion. Expressions for aerosol transport efficiency through ducts have been developed. The calculations are approximate, but have been used widely to compute sampling line losses and are known to give reasonable results in many cases. For these reasons, resuspension from duct surfaces requires a disturbance of some kind (mechanical shock, flow surges, or turbulent air burst), and the intensity of the disturbance affects both the concentration and the particle size of the resuspended aerosol.

PARTICLE MECHANICS

Steady Motion of Particles in Fluid—Stokes Law
As suggested earlier in the description of airflow in a cleanroom, there are cases when the particles have motion relative to the surrounding air. Understanding this motion is important for sampling of aerosols. The particle drag force in viscous flow is given by Stokes law:

$$F_D = 3\pi\eta V d_p \tag{2}$$

where F_D is the drag force on the particle, η the viscosity, V the particle velocity, and d_p the particle diameter (Fig. 3).

There are several assumptions underlying this equation: the fluid is incompressible, the particle is not near a wall, motion is constant, particle is a rigid sphere, and the fluid velocity at the surface of the particle is zero. The difference between the gravitational force and the drag force yields the sedimentation velocity. This is shown by:

$$F_D = F_g = mg \tag{3}$$

$$3\pi\eta V d_p = \frac{(\rho_p - \rho_g)\pi d_p^3 g}{6}$$
$$V_{TS} = \frac{\rho_p d_p^2 g}{18\eta} \tag{4}$$

where F_g is the force of gravity, m the mass of the particle, ρ_g the gas density, ρ_p the particle density, g the gravitational constant (980 cm/s/s), and V_{TS} the terminal sedimentation velocity (cm/s).

As mentioned above, one way to characterize irregular or nonspherical particles is to use the equivalent diameter concept. The settling velocity equation (4) has been used to determine an equivalent particle diameter. However, particle diameter, particle density, and shape are often unknown for a given observed settling velocity. The following particle diameters are defined (10):

$$V_{TS} = \frac{\rho_p d_e^2 g}{18\eta\chi} = \frac{\rho_b d_s^2 g}{18\eta} = \frac{\rho_0 d_a^2 g}{18\eta} \tag{5}$$

where d_e is the equivalent volume diameter, the diameter of a sphere having the same volume as the irregular particle; χ the dynamic shape factor, d_s Stokes diameter, the diameter of the sphere that has the same density and settling velocity as the irregular particle; and d_a the aerodynamic diameter, i.e., the diameter of the unit density ($\rho_p = 1$ g/cm^3) sphere that has the same settling velocity as the irregular particle.

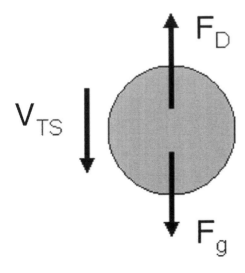

FIGURE 3 Force balance on a particle illustrating that the difference in drag and an external force such as gravity yields a net velocity.

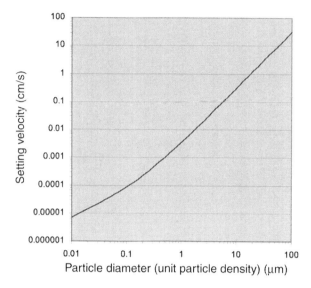

FIGURE 4 Particle settling velocity as a function of particle diameter. The particles are spherical with a particle density $= 1$ g/cm^3 in still air.

Aerodynamic diameter is a widely used descriptor of particles for which instruments using the inertial separation can be accurate. The aerodynamic diameter is also quite useful to describe processes which depend on particle inertia such as inhalation health effects, high-velocity filtration, impaction, cyclones, etc.

There are three observations with respect to Figure 4. (i) Particles larger than about 5 μm settle rapidly from the air and suspensions are unstable. (ii) Particles smaller than about 1 μm have vary small settling velocities and can be quite stable. (iii) Finally, the curve has a slight concave curvature due to deviation from the Stokes d_p^2 relationship for small particles. One of the assumptions of Stokes law is the velocity of the fluid at the surface of the particle surface is zero. However, as the size of the particles approach molecular dimensions, this assumption becomes less valid. In effect, the particles "slip" past the gas molecules to a greater extent than predicted than just with the Stokes law. Cunningham developed the first slip correction factors (10). The slip correction factor is given by:

$$C_c = 1 + \frac{\lambda}{d_p}\left[2.514 + 0.800 \ \exp\left(-0.55\frac{d_p}{\lambda}\right)\right] \tag{6}$$

where λ is the mean free path of the gas molecules.

In Figure 5, the slip correction is shown for standard conditions. The correction Equation (6) is semiempirical based on data taken over a range of particles and environmental conditions.

Particle Diffusion

Brownian motion is the movement of particles from collisions with surrounding molecules observed by Robert Brown in water suspensions of pollen. For particles less than 0.1 μm in diameter, diffusion caused by Brownian motion may be an important factor in predicting their behavior (10). Brownian motion will in effect move particles from regions of high concentration to low concentration. Particle diffusion is an important mechanism for the collection of Sub-0.1 μm particles in

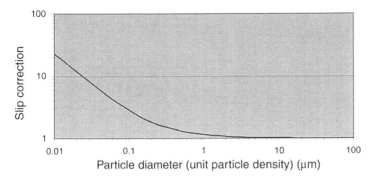

FIGURE 5 Slip correction as a function of particle diameter. The particles are assumed to be spherical.

air flowing through filters and tubes. The diffusion coefficient for aerosol particles is given by the Stokes–Einstein equation:

$$D = \frac{kTC_c}{3\pi\eta d_p} \tag{7}$$

where D is the diffusion coefficient and k Boltzmann's constant.

Figure 6 shows the inverse relationship of the diffusion coefficient with particle diameter in Equation (7).

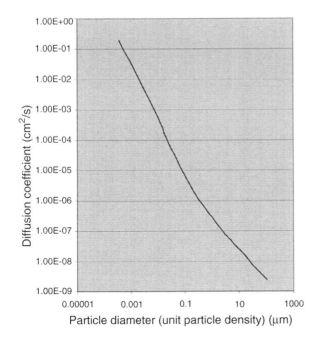

FIGURE 6 The diffusion coefficient as a function of particle diameter. The lower size limit of 0.00037 µm represents the diameter of an "air molecule."

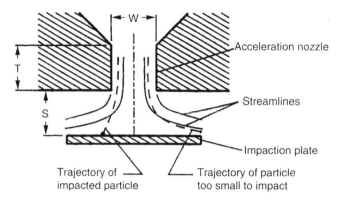

FIGURE 7 Illustration of an impactor showing the position of nozzle and impaction surface. *Abbreviation*: W is the width of the acceleration nozzle, T is the depth of the nozzle, S is the distance from the nozzle to the impaction plate. *Source*: From Ref. 32.

Inertial Effects (Unsteady Flow Conditions)

Particles of sufficient size will exhibit inertial effects, which cause a deviation from airflow streamlines. Example of this occurs when particles are accelerated in a nozzle and the air jet directed at a surface as shown in Figure 7. Impactors are often used to capture particles by directing against a collection surface for subsequent analysis (29). Impactors are often used with media for bioaerosol sampling (30) with appropriate corrections (31). These are often called sieve or silt samplers, examples are Anderson sampler and slit to agar samplers. In general, the greater the jet velocity, the smaller the particle that can be collected. However, the jet velocity is limited by sonic velocity. Also high-velocity jets may blow-off of the particles from the collection surface. Therefore, for most conventional impactors, the limit for particle collection is about 0.3 μm. Impactors have been developed using very small jet diameters and low pressure to allow collection of particles smaller than 0.1 μm (32).

The efficiency of an impactor depends on the Stokes number. The Stokes number is defined as:

$$Stk = \rho_p d_p^2 U C_c / 9\eta D_j \tag{8}$$

where ρ_p is the density of the particle, d_p the particle diameter, U the velocity through the jet, C_c the Cunningham correction factor, n the viscosity of gas, and D_j the diameter of hole forming the jet.

The collecting efficiency can be computed with fluid dynamic simulations of an impactor (32). In practice, the impactor is calibrated to obtain the appropriate collection efficiencies.

In Figure 8, impactor collection efficiency is shown for various collection surfaces. Theory assumes that a particle touching the surface of the substrate is captured. In practice, particles may bounce or can be resuspended from the surface. In the extremes are an oiled surface and bare surfaces. Fiber filter mats have used as collection substrates to reduce particle bounce. As seen in the figure, the efficiency of a filter mat is midway between the bare and the oiled surfaces. For some regions of Stokes number, the collection substrate may act like a filter of the air flowing parallel along the collection surface. Usually bounce is not a problem for microorganism sampling because the agar is fairly sticky and the jet velocity

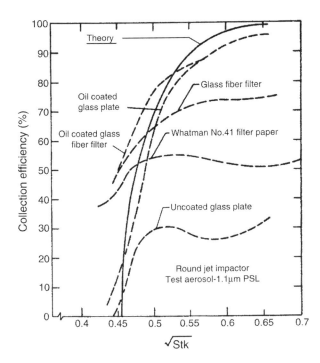

FIGURE 8 Effect of collection surface on impactor cutoff curve. *Source*: From Ref. 33. Reprinted with permission of the University Press of Florida. *Abbreviation*: PSL, polystyrene latex.

is low to prevent damage to the organism. Other problems include overloading with particles or excessive sampling times, which will dry the media.

Other External Forces
Under some circumstances, a suspended particle may be moved appreciably by external gradients such as light, heat, and electrical charge.

Electrical
Particles usually have an electrical charge resulting from a wide range of mechanisms during formation and transport. Charged particles will follow Coulombs law and will be attracted to other particles and surfaces of opposite charge and will be repelled by identical polarity. Naturally occurring particles typically will be charged (34).

Thermal
Dark spots near the wall near an old-fashioned radiator for interior heating is a common example. Particles move from high temperatures to low temperatures (along the temperature gradient). The effect is strongly dependent on particle diameter with the greatest effect found for the smallest particles (35).

Light
Normally under normal ambient light illumination and ambient atmospheric pressures found in a cleanroom, the effects of light on particles are insignificant. However, under conditions of either/or high intensities such as that generated by a laser or low pressure, light forces can be significant. There are two mechanisms: the light heats the particle and the thermal gradient causes motion either in the direction

of the light or away depending on the refractive index of the particle or in some cases the momentum from photons can cause motions away from the light (36).

FILTRATION

Air filtration is vital to the central purpose of cleanroom to create an environment with acceptably low particle contamination. The heating, ventilation, and air conditioning system contains general ventilation and high-efficiency filters. The cleanroom itself typically uses ceiling HEPA filters. Small filters may also used in samplers to collect air samples of particles.

Filter Materials

A wide variety of filters are available. Filters are designed to remove particles with the least pressure drop. Filters have been made from various kinds of polymers, glass fibers, porous membranes, fibrillated polymeric films, and porous metals. A fibrous filter medium used for HEPA filtration is shown in Figure 9.

The goal in selecting filters is to maintain the highest flow rate, lowest pressure drop, and lowest particle penetration. The penetration is the outlet concentration divided by the inlet concentration. The efficiency of a filter is defined in terms of the fractional penetration of particles:

$$\text{Efficiency}(\%) = (1 - \text{penetration}) \times 100 \tag{9}$$

Fractional penetration is the ratio of the outlet concentration divided by the inlet concentration at a range of particle of varying sizes.

Fibrous filters collect particles primarily by the following mechanisms: interception, inertial impaction, diffusion, and electrostatic attraction as illustrated in Figure 10. Detailed filtration theory and the importance of the collection mechanisms have been reviewed (37,38).

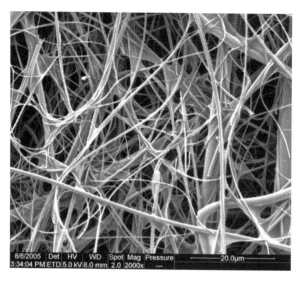

FIGURE 9   Micrograph of typical HEPA fibrous filter media (2000x). *Source*: From Dr. Howard J. Walls.

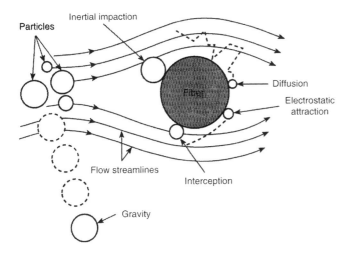

FIGURE 10 Illustration of the mechanisms responsible for particle collection in fibrous filters.

Interception occurs when a particle comes into contact and sticks to the fiber while following the airflow streamline. This mechanism depends on the ratio of the particle diameter to the fiber diameter and is effective for particles larger than 1 mm. The physical parameters of importance include particle diameter, fiber diameter, filter packing density, and depth.

Collection by diffusion is effective for particles smaller than 0.1 μm. This collection mechanism results from the random Brownian motion driving the particles to the fiber. It is dependent on the ratio of the particle diffusion coefficient to the air velocity through the filter. The physical parameters of importance are particle diameter, fiber diameter, air velocity, filter packing density, and depth.

Inertial deposition occurs when a particle deviates from the flow streamline from its inertia as the air flows around the fiber and contacts the fiber. This mechanism is most effective on particles larger than a few tenths of a micron because it utilizes the inertia of the particle and works best in systems with high air velocities. The physical properties of importance include particle mass, air velocity, and fiber diameter, particle phase that may affect particle bounce, filter packing density, and depth.

Electrostatic attraction occurs when the particle and/or fiber has an electrostatic charge. Electrostatic particle collection mechanisms are important for three applications: (i) Active electrostatic systems use corona charging of the particles and/or use an electric field on a filter mat. A number of different electrostatically augmented systems have been available for at least 50 years (39). (ii) Tribogeneration by the passage of air over dielectric fibers. (iii) Permanently electrostatically charged fibers. The Hansen filter for respirators developed in the 1930s used triboelectrically charged resin in wool filters (40). Modern permanent electrostatic filters use polymer fibers that have been processed with corona discharge or fibrillated sheets of electret material to provide a permanent charge on the fibers. These filters have enhanced efficiency until the charges are covered or shielded by particles (41). The physical parameters of importance include particle charge, fiber charge, particle mass, air velocity, filter packing density, and depth.

In Figure 11, particles larger than 0.1 μm are collected predominately by interception. For low-efficiency filters with high face velocities, impaction may be

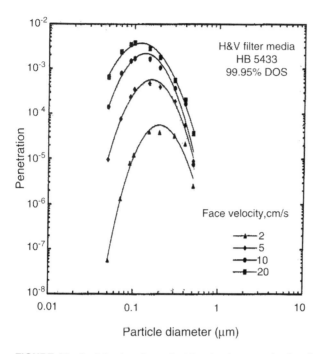

FIGURE 11 Particle size–dependent fractional penetration for cleanroom filters. *Source*: From Ref. 42. *Abbreviations*: DOS, dioctylsebacate; H&V, Hollingsworth and Vose.

significant. Collection by diffusion is predominant below 0.1 μm. The most penetrating particle diameter is at the point in the filtration curve where the diffusion and interception mechanisms are least effective. The most penetrating particle diameter depends on the face velocity, porosity, and fiber diameter. The particle penetration of the filter tends to increase and the most penetrating diameter tends to be reduced because the shorter residence time in the media reduces the effectiveness of diffusion. Typically the most penetrating diameter is from 0.1 to 0.5 μm depending on the type of filter. High-efficiency filters are normally tested at the most penetrating particle diameter (43–45). As microorganisms of interest have larger diameters than the most penetrating particle diameter, the penetration of microorganisms is lower than the penetration of the most penetrating diameter (46). The filtration efficiency and the pressure drop will increase with time as the filter collects particles (47).

AIR SAMPLING IN CLEANROOMS

Air sampling in cleanrooms is an essential activity. Understanding the physical properties of particles, their sources, and their behavior is key to developing a good, effective sampling program. Knowing where to sample in a cleanroom can prevent many problems by identifying problems early.

Sampling via Nozzles or Inlets

The sampling of the air from a cleanroom involves aspirating air from ambient air through a nozzle. Ideally, the particles in the air would enter the sample nozzle

ISOAXIAL SAMPLING

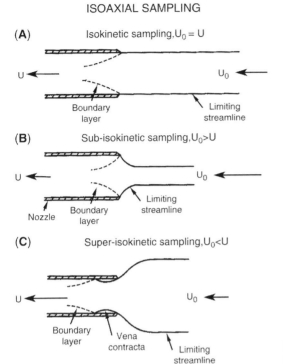

(A) Isokinetic sampling,$U_0 = U$

U ◀— U_0 ◀—

Boundary layer

Limiting streamline

(B) Sub-isokinetic sampling,$U_0>U$

U ◀— U_0 ◀—

Nozzle Boundary layer Limiting streamline

(C) Super-isokinetic sampling,$U_0<U$

U ◀— U_0 ◀—

Boundary layer Vena contracta Limiting streamline

FIGURE 12 Illustration of isokinetic sampling flow. *Source*: From Ref. 48.

without separation of particle by size from inertial effects or deposition of the particles inside the nozzle or tubing. The preferred sampling approach is to match the flow velocity in the inlet with the velocity in the ambient air. The effect of mismatched air velocity in affecting particle concentration is shown in Figure 12. Sample biases tend to be caused by inertial effects found in larger particles. The instrument may under sample the large particles if the velocity in the inlet is much larger than the surrounding air. In this case, small particles from an area of approaching air larger than the area of the nozzle are drawn into the sample. If the air velocity at the inlet is less than the surrounding air, the larger particles would be enriched. The effective area of the nozzle for fine particles is smaller than the area of the nozzle, whereas the larger particles because of their inertia will continue on their preestablished trajectories enriching the sample. The entry of particle into a sampling tube is dependent on several parameters. These include (*i*) airflow velocity (and turbulence) in the surrounding air, (*ii*) size and flow velocity of the sampling inlet, and (*iii*) the angle of the sampling nozzle with respect to the airflow direction. For example, if the particles are sampled by a nozzle at right angles to the direction of airflow, the large particles would be thrown away from the nozzle by the change in airflow direction.

In Figure 13, the concentration changes, with ambient flow velocity U_o and sample flow velocity U ratio as a parameter, are shown as a function of the square root of the stokes number (49). The relative angle θ of the nozzle to the ambient air flow direction; perfect alignment occurs when θ is zero. The square root of the Stokes number is proportional to particle size. Therefore, for very small particles

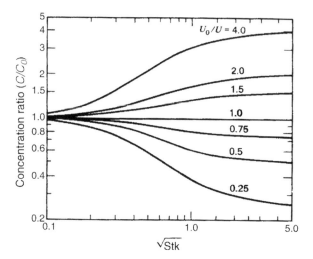

FIGURE 13 Concentration ration versus the square root of Stokes number for several values of velocity ration, $\theta = 0$, based on Durham and Lundgren empirical results. *Source*: From Refs. 10 and 49.

the air velocities are unimportant. However, when the square root of the Stokes number is larger than 1, the velocity ratio can be quite important.

Sample Transport Through Tubes

After entry into the sampling tube, the particles are transported through the tubing to the sampler. Mechanisms affecting the particles are the same as described above: (*i*) gravitational sedimentation (*ii*), inertial deposition in elbows (*iii*), turbulent deposition (*iv*), loss by diffusion, and possibly (*v*) electrostatic deposition on surfaces. To reduce deposition from electrostatic effects, conducting tubing material should be used. From a practical standpoint, tubing as short as possible should be used. Also, large radius bends with radius of curvature four times the tubing diameter should be used if bends are needed. Also expansions and contractions of the tubing diameter or in fittings should be avoided. The flow velocity is also important affecting residence time in the tube important for gravitational sedimentation, velocity in the turns, and turbulence. Turbulence in the tubing is determined by computation of the Reynolds number:

$$Re = \frac{DU\rho_g}{\mu} \tag{10}$$

where D is the tubing diameter. When Re is less than 2000, the flow is laminar. When Re is greater than 4000, the flow is turbulent.

Typically, flow rates are selected to produce sufficient velocity for turbulent flow but low enough to minimize deposition in bends. In Figure 14, transport efficiency (the fraction of particles penetrating the tube) shows the effects of tubing length for laminar and turbulent flows.

The transport efficiency is shown in Figure 14 as a function of aerodynamic particle diameter with tubing length and Reynolds number as parameters. These results were computed using Deposition 4.0 developed by McFarland (50). The most important parameter is the particle diameter. The next most important is

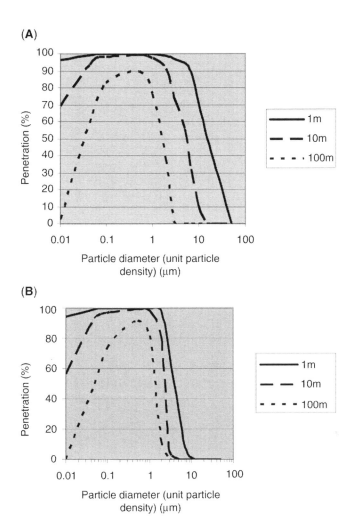

(A)

(B)

FIGURE 14 Tubing length. (**A**) Penetration of particles through a circular tube 12.7 mm (1/2 in) in diameter with tubing length as a parameter in laminar flow. The flow rate was 10 lpm and the $Re = 275$. (**B**) Penetration of particles through a circular tube 6.35 mm (1/4 in) in diameter with tubing length as a parameter in turbulent flow. The flow rate was 30 lpm and the $Re = 5000$.

the tubing length. Turbulence enhances deposition for particles larger than 10 mm as shown by comparing the deposition in Figure 14A and B.

CLEANROOM DYNAMICS

Operational States

As described earlier, cleanroom conditions can be described by its operational states: (*i*) as-built, (*ii*) standby, and (*iii*) operational. The particles in the cleanroom will depend on these states. For example, in the operational state the effects of personnel and process equipment will become significant.

Particle Bursts/Transport

It has been observed (25) that long-term measurements in operational cleanroom yield steady particle concentrations with occasional short, random, relatively high concentration of particles or "particle bursts." These busts of particles have been related to specific processes.

Effect of Activity

The measurement of particle size distribution over a wide range of particle diameter and integrated over particle bursts during operational states is difficult to perform. Ensor et al. (51) described the use of an array of condensation nuclei counters with diffusion batteries to limit the particles to a specific size range. Diffusion batteries contain a series of screens selected so that the small particles are collected and the larger particles pass through the device. Six condensation nuclei counters and two optical counters were used. The sampling array can be used to directly obtain the "larger than or equal to" cumulative particle size distribution curves used in cleanroom standards. The at-rest cumulative "larger than or equal to" specific particle diameter curve in Figure 15A shows the source of the particles are particles from outside penetrating the air filters in the 0.1–0.3 μm particle size range. During the work day, when the cleanroom is in operation, both very small and large particles are introduced into the air as indicated by the straight curve in Figure 15B . It was observed that particle counts in a cleanroom rise during periods of activity in the cleanroom.

During the at-rest or inactive state, the size distribution in the cleanroom is defined by the filter particle size-dependent efficiency. If the filter penetration curve as presented in Figure 11 is converted to a cumulative curve, the particle size distribution curve observed at rest in Figure 15A will be predicted. The implication is that in the cleanroom studied the size distribution during nights without activity that the particles results mainly from atmospheric ambient air particles that are not collected by the filter. Because of the low penetration or high particle collection, the concentration within the cleanroom is orders of magnitudes lower than the outside air. When the room is active, both large and small particles are introduced into the cleanroom from internal sources as shown in Figure 15B. The sources of particles described earlier could all influence the particle concentrations. As this was an electronic cleanroom, it is expected that the fine particles less than 0.5 μm were caused by thermal generation by the furnaces or wafer coating operations. The larger particles greater than 0.5 μm were likely caused by emissions from personnel or resuspension from the floors (52–54).

Surface Deposition

Deposition of particles to surfaces in the cleanroom is important for two reasons: critical work surfaces may be contaminated by particles deposited from the air and particles may be monitored with witness plates or exposed slides. However, particle deposition is particle size-dependent. This means that sampling surfaces either by wipe sampling or witness plates will have a bias due to the differences in deposition velocity.

$$\text{Deposition velocity} = \frac{\text{Concentration}(\#/m^3)}{\text{flux}(\#/m^2/\text{sec})} \tag{11}$$

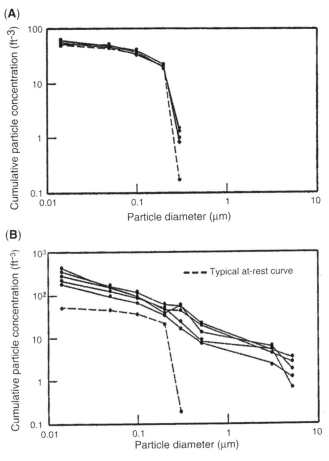

FIGURE 15   (**A**) Cleanroom particle size distribution during an at-rest state measured at night while no operators were present. (**B**) Cleanroom particle size distribution during an operational state measured during a normal workday. *Source*: From Ref. 51.

Ideally deposition velocity in the above equation is measured by measuring the concentration above the surface while measuring the flux or the number of particle per unit area. In the large particle limit, the deposition velocity equals to the sedimentation velocity. However, as the particle diameter is reduced, other forces, such as turbulence, electrical forces, Brownian diffusion, and phoretic forces from temperature gradients, become important and will affect deposition velocity (55–58). Brownian diffusion increases the deposition of submicron particles in a manner similar to that described earlier for filtration and deposition in tubing. Computations of deposition velocities in a unidirectional flow cleanroom are shown in Figure 16 (54). The deposition velocity is a combination of settling velocity as shown in Figure 4 and diffusion following the trend in Figure 6. The higher the deposition velocity, the more likely the particle will be deposited on the surface. The minimum in the particle deposition curve means that particles in the 0.1–1 μm range are relatively stable in the air. These theoretical curves for deposition are reasonably predictive of actual deposition rates (59).

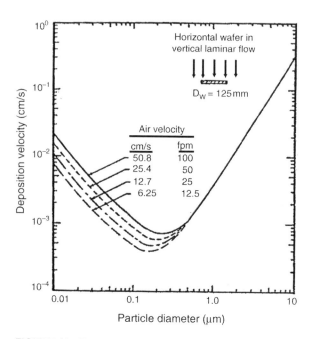

FIGURE 16 Particle deposition onto a 125-mm round horizontal surface in a unidirectional flow cleanroom. *Source*: From Ref. 55.

SUMMARY

The behavior of particles in cleanrooms starts with sources of the particles and transport within the cleanroom. The sources may be from outside the cleanroom, processes or equipment within the cleanroom, and personnel operating the cleanroom. As an approximation, the particles will follow the air flowing in the cleanroom. However, particles may deviate from the bulk airflow from gravitational sedimentation, inertial effects if the air suddenly changes direction, Brownian diffusion, and other outside forces such as electrostatics, thermal, and light.

Solid particles are rarely perfect spheres. Often equivalent diameters rather than physical diameter are used to describe the particle. The equivalent particle diameter often results from the method of measurement. The particle size is the primary variable in determining particle behavior.

The mechanisms of particle generation include resuspension, spraying of liquids, combustion, or thermal processes.

There may be significant biases when sampling aerosols. For example, the entry of particles depends on the relative velocity within the nozzle and the ambient air and orientation of the tube to the airflow velocity. If the sample nozzle is not aligned with the direction of airflow, the size distribution may be enriched or depleted in large particles, and deposition within the nozzle may be increased. Particles may also be lost in tubing by gravitational settling and deposition on bends.

In an operating cleanroom, the particle size distribution depends on the level of activity.

REFERENCES

1. ISO 14644-4. Cleanrooms and Associated Controlled Environments—Part 4: Design, Construction and Startup.
2. ISO 14644-1. Cleanrooms and Associated Controlled Environments—Part 1: Classification of Air Cleanliness.
3. ISO 14644-2. Cleanrooms and Associated Controlled Environments—Part 2: Specifications for Testing and Monitoring to Prove Continued Compliance with ISO 14644-1.
4. ISO 14698-1. Cleanrooms and Associated Controlled Environments—Part 1: Biocontamination Control, General Principles and Methods.
5. ISO 14698-2. Cleanrooms and Associated Controlled Environments—Part 2: Biocontamination Control, Evaluation, and Interpretation of Biocontamination Data.
6. Yamamoto T, Donovan RP, Ensor DS. Model study for optimization of cleanroom airflows. J Environ Sci 1988; 31(6):24–29.
7. Yamamoto T. Airflow modeling and particle control by vertical laminar flow. In: Donovan RP, ed. Particle Control for Semiconductor Manufacturing. New York: Marcel Dekker, 1990:301–323.
8. Fitzner K. Particle movement in cleanrooms with laminar flow. In: Proceedings of the Ninth ICCCS, Los Angeles, 1988:657–662.
9. Ensor DS. Particle size distributions. In: Donovan RP, ed. Particle Control for Semiconductor Manufacturing. New York: Marcel Dekker, 1990:27–45.
10. Hinds WC. Aerosol Technology. New York: Wiley, 1982.
11. Sem GJ. The dynamics of aerosols in cleanroom environments: implication for monitoring and control of airborne particles and their sources. In: Donovan RP, ed. Particle Control for Semiconductor Manufacturing. New York: Marcel Dekker, 1990:143–157.
12. Dixon AM. Guidelines for cleanroom management and discipline. In: Tolliver DL, ed. Handbook of Contamination Control in Microelectronics. Park Ridge: Noyes Publications, 1988:136–152.
13. ISO 14644-5. Cleanrooms and Associated Controlled Environments—Part 5: Operations.
14. Reeks MW, Hall D. Deposition and resuspension of gas-borne particles in recirculating turbulent flows. J Fluids Eng 1988; 110:165–171.
15. Jurcik B, Wang H-C. The modeling of particle resuspension in turbulent flow. J Aerosol Sci 1991; 22(suppl 1):S149–S152.
16. Ziskind G, Fichman M, Gutfinger C. Resuspension of particles from surfaces to turbulent flows—review and analysis. J Aerosol Sci. 1995; 26:613–644.
17. Lake E, Watanabe N, Goto H, Kitano M. The effect of sedimentary particles on floors in non-unidirectional airflow cleanrooms. In: Proceedings of Institute of Environmental Sciences and Technology, Phoenix, 1998:581–587.
18. Foarde K, Berry M. A comparison of biocontaminant levels associated with hard vs. carpet floors in nonproblem schools: results of a year long study. J Expo Anal Environ Epidemiol Macher JM 2004; 14(suppl 1):S41–S48.
19. Whyte W, Bailey PV. Particle dispersion in relation to clothing. J Environ Sci 1989; 32(2):43–49.
20. IEST RP-CC 003.3. Garment system considerations for cleanrooms and other controlled environments. Institute of Environmental Science and Technology, Rolling Meadows, 2003.
21. Ensor DS, Elion JM, Eudy J. The size distribution of particles released by garments during Helmke drum tests. J Inst Environ Sci Technol 2001; 44(4):24–27.

22. Elion JM, Ensor DS, Berndt C, et al. Improving the repeatability and reproducibility of the Helmke drum test method. J Inst Environ Sci Technol 2001; 44(4):28–32.
23. IEST RP-CC 0026. Cleanroom Operations. Rolling Meadows: Institute of Environmental Science and Technology, 2004.
24. Donovan RP, Locke BR, Ensor DS. Test method for measuring aerosol particle emission rates from cleanroom equipment. Microcontamination 1987; 5(10):36–39, 60–63.
25. Viner AS. Predicted and measured cleanroom contamination. In: Donovan RP, ed. Particle Control for Semiconductor Manufacturing. New York: Marcel Dekker, 1990:129–141.
26. Lacey J. The aerobiology of conidial fungi. In: Gary TC, Bryce K, eds. Biology of Conidial Fungi. New York: Academic Press, 1981:373–416.
27. Foarde KK, VanOsdell DW, Ensor DS. Entrainment and transport of bioaerosols for ventilation ducts. In: Proceedings of ICCCS 14th International Symposium on Contamination Control. Phoenix, April 26–May 1, 1998:459–465.
28. Zimon AD. Adhesion of Dust and Powder. New York: Plenum Press, 1980.
29. Lodge JP, Chan TL, eds. Cascade Impactor. Akron: American Industrial Hygiene Association, 1986.
30. Macher J, ed. Bioaerosols: Assessment and Control. American Conference of Governmental Industrial Hygienists. Cincinnati, 1999.
31. Macher JM. Positive-hole correction of multiple-jet impactors for collecting viable microorganisms. Am Indus Hygiene Assoc J 1989; 50:561–568.
32. Marple VA, Rubow KL, Olson BA. Inertial, gravitational, centrifugal, and thermal collection techniques. In: Willeke K, Baron P, eds. Aerosol Measurement. New York: Van Nostrand Reinhold, 1993:206–232.
33. Marple VA, Willeke K. Inertial impactors. In: Lundren DA, Harris FS, Marlow WH, Lippmann M, Clark WE, Durham MD, eds. Aerosol Measurement. Gainesville: University of Florida Press, 1979:90–107.
34. Donovan RP. Particle deposition data: room air ionization as a control method. In: Donovan RP, ed. Particle Control for Semiconductor Manufacturing. New York: Marcel Dekker, 1990:325–340.
35. Nazaroff WW, Cass GR. Mass-transport aspects of pollutant removal at indoor surfaces. Environ Int 1989; 15:567–584.
36. Preining O. Photophoresis. In: Davies CN, ed. Aerosol Science. New York: Academic Press, 1966:111–135.
37. Kirsch AA, Stechkina IB. The theory of aerosol filtration with fibrous filters. In: Shaw DT, ed. Fundamentals of Aerosol Science. New York: Wiley, 1978:165–256.
38. Ensor DS, Donovan RP. Aerosol filtration technology. In: Tolliver DL, ed. Handbook of Contamination Control in Microelectronics. Park Ridge: Noyes Publications, 1988:1–63.
39. Donovan RP, VanOsdell DW. Electrical enhancement of fabric filtration. In: Cheremisinoff NP, ed. Encyclopedia of Fluid Flow. Houston: Gulf Publishing Co., 1986:1331–1359.
40. Davies CN. Air Filtration. New York: Academic Press, 1973.
41. Romay FT, Liu BYH, Chae S-J. Experimental study of electrostatic capture mechanism in commercial electret filters. Aerosol Sci Technol 1998; 28:224–234.
42. Dhaniyala S, Liu BYH. Investigations of particle penetration in fibrous filters. J Inst Environ Sci Technol 1999; 42(1):32–40.
43. IEST RP-CC 001.3. HEPA and ULPA filters. Rolling Meadows: Institute of Environmental Science and Technology, 1993.

44. IEST RP-CC 002.2. Unidirectional flow clean air devices. Rolling Meadows: Institute of Environmental Science and Technology, 1999.
45. IEST RP-CC 007.1. Testing ULPA Filters. Rolling Meadows: Institute of Environmental Science and Technology, 1992.
46. Decker HM, Buchanan LM, Hall LB, Goddard KR. Air filtration of microbial particles. Am J Public Health 1962; 53:1982–1988.
47. Thomas D, Contal P, Renaudin V, Penicot P, Leclere D, Vendel J. Modelling pressure drop in HEPA filters during dynamic filtration. J Aerosol Sci 1999; 30:235–246.
48. Brockmann JE. Sampling and transport of aerosols. In: Willeke K, Baron PA, eds. Aerosol Measurement. New York: Van Nostrand Reinhold, 1993:77–111.
49. Durham MD, Lundgren DH. Evaluation of aerosol aspiration efficiency as a function of Stokes number, velocity ration, and nozzle angle. J Aerosol Sci 1980; 11:179–188.
50. McFarland AR. Deposition Version 4.0. College Station, TX: Aerosol Technology Laboratory, Department of Mechanical Engineering, Texas A&M University.
51. Ensor DS, Viner AS, Johnson EW, Donovan EW, Keady PB, Weyrauch KJ. Measurement of ultrafine aerosol particle size distributions at low concentrations by parallel arrays of a diffusion battery and a condensation nucleus counter in series. J Aerosol Sci 1989; 20(4):471–475.
52. Ensor DS, Donovan RP, Locke BR. Particle size distributions in cleanrooms. J Environ Sci 1987; 30(6):44–49.
53. Donovan RP, Locke BR, Ensor DS, Osburn CM. The case for incorporating condensation nuclei counters into a standard for air quality. Microcontamination 1984; 8:(12), 39–44.
54. Liu BYH, Lee JW, Pui DYH, Ahn KH, Gilbert SL. Performance of a laboratory cleanroom. J Environ Sci 1998; 30(5):22–25.
55. Liu BYH, Ahn K. Particle deposition on semiconductor wafers. Aerosol Sci Technol 1987; 6(3):215–224.
56. Nazaroff WW, Cass GR. Particle deposition from a natural convection flow onto a vertical isothermal flat plate. J Aerosol Sci 1987; 18:445–455.
57. Fissan HJ, Turner JR. Electrostatic effects in particle deposition onto product surfaces. In: Proceedings of the ICCCS, Los Angeles, 1988:400–404.
58. Turner JR, Liguras DK, Fissan HJ. Cleanroom applications of particle deposition from stagnation flow: electrostatics effects. J Aerosol Sci 1989; 20(4):403–417.
59. Wu JJ, Miller RJ, Cooper DW, Flynn JF, Delson DJ. Deposition of submicron aerosol particles during integrated circuit manufacturing: experiments. J Environ Sci 1989; 27(1):27–45.

2 The Application of the New International Standards Organization Cleanroom Standards

Richard A. Matthews

- The International Standards
- Guidelines
- Working Groups
- Documents and Their Titles
- ISO Project Stages and Associated Documents
- Specific Information on Each Standard
    - *ISO 14644-1 Classification of Air Cleanliness (18 Pages)*
    - *ISO 14644-2—Specifications for Testing and Monitoring to Prove Continued Compliance with ISO 14644-1 (7 Pages)*
    - *ISO 14644-3 Test Methods (62 Pages)*
    - *ISO 14644-4—Design, Construction, and Startup (51 Pages)*
    - *ISO 14644-5 Operations (44 Pages)*
    - *ISO 14644-6—Vocabulary (21 Pages)*
    - *ISO 14644-7—Separative Devices (Clean Air Hoods, Glove Boxes, Isolators, and Mini Environments) (52 Pages)*
    - *ISO 14644-8—Classification of Airborne Molecular Contamination (22 Pages)*
    - *ISO 14698-1 (32 Pages) and ISO 14698-2 (11 Pages) Biocontamination Control*
- Summary
- Reference

2 The Application of the New International Standards Organization Cleanroom Standards

Richard A. Matthews
Filtration Technology, Inc., Greensboro, North Carolina, U.S.A.

THE INTERNATIONAL STANDARDS

In 1992, at the instigation of the Institute of Environmental Sciences and Technology (IEST), the American National Standards Institute (ANSI) petitioned the International Standards Organization (ISO) to create a new technical committee, "Clean Rooms and Associated Controlled Environments." This new technical committee, ISO/TC 209, was formally established in May, 1993. The importance of this endeavor is underscored by the fact that currently there are over 50,000 cleanrooms worldwide, with an annual economic impact in excess of $1 trillion.

The ANSI is responsible for participation in those technical areas of work where the United States' interests have dictated support. ANSI then looks to a nonprofit organization that develops standards in a particular technology area to determine the United States' position in a similar international standardization activity. The IEST is the body of choice for the activity of ISO/TC 209.

The mission of this technical committee is to develop a series of international standards for cleanrooms and associated controlled environments, encompassing standardization of equipment, facilities, and operational methods. ISO/TC 209 defines procedural limits, operational limits, and testing procedures to achieve desired attributes to minimize contamination.

Topics of interest are nonviable particles, viable particles, surface cleanliness, airflow patterns and velocities, room infiltration leakage, personnel procedures, personnel clothing, equipment preparation, and other topics related to optimizing cleanroom operations. Currently there are 19 voting members, designated as "P" members, 20 nonvoting "O" members, and 5 formal liaison groups (Table 1).

GUIDELINES

These are the general guidelines established for ISO/TC 209 operations:

1. Do not define cleanrooms by user-specific applications.
2. Do nothing that causes a major economic impact to a specific nation.
3. Do not classify cleanrooms by microbial limits.
4. Standardize criteria for cleanrooms and related environments.
5. Eliminate trade barriers.
6. Consensus vote for all final drafts.
7. Recognize that ISO standards are not mandatory.

TABLE 1   ISO/TC 209 Member Nations and Liaison Groups

"P" Voting nations	"O" Observer nations
Australia	Argentina
Belgium	Barbados
Brazil	Bulgaria
China	Cuba
Denmark	Czech Republic
Finland	Egypt
France	Hungary
Germany	India
Italy	Ireland
Japan	Jamaica
Republic of Korea	Malaysia
Netherlands	Mexico
Norway	Philippines
Portugal	Poland
Russian Federation	Saudi Arabia
Sweden	Serbia and Montenegro
Switzerland	South Africa
United Kingdom	Thailand
United States	Turkey, Ukraine

Liaison groups
International Confederation of Contamination Control Societies
ISO/TC 146 (Air quality)
ISO/IC 198 (Sterilization of health-care products)
ISO/TC 229 (Nanotechnology)
CEN/TC 243 (Cleanroom technology)

WORKING GROUPS

In accordance with ISO procedures, all work is performed in working groups. Each voting member country can send two delegates to each group. Currently, there are nine working groups. The governorship of each working group is assigned to a voting nation (Table 2).

TABLE 2   ISO/TC 209 Working Groups

Number	Title	Convenor nation
1	Classes of air cleanliness	United Kingdom
2	Biocontamination	United Kingdom
3	Test methods	Japan
4	Design and construction	Germany
5	Operations	United States
6	Vocabulary	Switzerland
7	Separative devices	United States
8	Molecular contamination	United Kingdom
9	Clean surfaces	Switzerland

DOCUMENTS AND THEIR TITLES

14644-1	Classification of Air Cleanliness
14644-2	Specifications for Testing and Monitoring to Prove Continued Compliance with ISO 14644-1
14644-3	Test Methods
14644-4	Design and Construction
14644-5	Cleanroom Operations
14644-6	Vocabulary
14644-7	Separative Devices
14644-8	Molecular Contamination
14698-1	Biocontamination—General Principles
14698-2	Biocontamination—Evaluation and Interpretation of Biocontamination Data

ISO PROJECT STAGES AND ASSOCIATED DOCUMENTS

Project stage	Name	Abbreviation	Comment
Preliminary stage	Preliminary Work Item	PWI	First definition of work to be accomplished
Proposal stage activity	New Work Item Proposal	NP	Time-specific activity (must complete working draft within 6 months of NP)
Preparatory stage	Working Drafts	WD	Time-specific activity (must complete CD within 12 months of NP)
Committee stage	Committee Drafts	CD	Requires comment by national standards bodies within 3 to 6 months
Inquiry stage	Draft International Standard	DIS	Requires comment and vote by national standards bodies and P members within 5 months
Approval stage	Final Draft International Standard	FDIS	Incorporates changes from DIS and formal P member vote within 2 months
Publication stage	International Standard	ISO	Automatic publication within 2 months of FDIS vote

SPECIFIC INFORMATION ON EACH STANDARD

ISO 14644-1 Classification of Air Cleanliness (18 Pages)

The scope of this standard published in 1999 covers the classification of air cleanliness in cleanrooms and associated controlled environments exclusively in terms of concentration of airborne particles (Table 3).

Only particle populations having cumulative distributions based on threshold (lower limits) sizes ranging from 0.1 to 5.0 μm are considered for classification purposes. This standard is divided into the mandatory section called the normative

TABLE 3 Selected Airborne Particulate Cleanliness Classes for Cleanrooms

ISO Classification number	Maximum concentration limits (particles/m^3 of air)					
	$\geq 0.1\,\mu m$	$\geq 0.2\,\mu m$	$\geq 0.3\,\mu m$	$\geq 0.5\,\mu m$	$\geq 1\,\mu m$	$\geq 5.0\,\mu m$
ISO Class 1	10	2				
ISO Class 2	100	24	10	4		
ISO Class 3	1000	237	102	35	8	
ISO Class 4	10,000	2370	1020	352	83	
ISO Class 5	100,000	23,700	10,200	3520	832	29
ISO Class 6	1,000,000	237,000	102,000	35,200	8320	293
ISO Class 7				352,000	83,200	2930
ISO Class 8				3,520,000	832,000	29,300
ISO Class 9				35,200,000	8,320,000	293,000

and annexes, of which some are normative and others informative. Within the normative sections are the mandatory criteria. These include:

- Classes of air cleanliness
- Mathematical method for determining air cleanliness classification
- Determination of air cleanliness classification using a discrete particle counter (DPC)
- Statistical treatment of particle concentration data
- You must specify and report:

  1. ISO Class
  2. Occupancy state
  3. Particle size or sizes

The particle classification of air in a cleanroom or a clean zone is defined in one or more of these occupancy states—"as built," "at rest," or "operational."

- "As built" is a condition where the installation is complete, with all the services connected and functioning, but contains no production equipment, materials, or personnel.
- "At rest" is a condition where the installation is complete with the equipment installed but personnel are not present.
- "Operational" is a condition where the installation is functioning, equipment is running, and personnel are present.

The airborne classification is based upon the maximum permitted concentration of particles for each particle size. This is based on the following formula:

$$C_n = 10^N \times \frac{(0.1)^{2.08}}{D}$$

where C_n is the maximum permitted concentration in particles per cubic meter of air of airborne particles that are equal to or larger than the considered particle size. N is the ISO classification number, which shall not exceed a value of 9. (Intermediate ISO classifications may be specified with 0.1, the smallest permitted increment of N.) D is the considered particle size in micrometers. 0.1 is a constant with the dimension of micrometers. Annex D provides examples of classification calculations.

However, provisions are made to quantify particles smaller than 0.1 μm. These are called ultrafine particles and may be quantified with a U descriptor. Conversely, particles larger than 5.0 μm are called macroparticles and may be quantified with an M descriptor. U and M descriptors are not used in classification of air cleanliness, but they may be used for defining acceptable and/or measurable levels of nonclassified air cleanliness. Found in Annex B is the determination of particle cleanliness classifications using a discrete-particle counting, light- scattering instrument. To derive the minimum number of sampling points, the equation is

$$N_L = \sqrt{A}$$

where N_L is the minimum number of sampling locations. A is the area of the cleanroom in square meters.

For example, a cleanroom measuring 30 ft × 40 ft has an area of 1200 square feet. This converts to 111.5 m². The square root of 111.5 is 10.56 rounded to 11 sampling locations.

Annex B does allow for the establishment of a single sample location. To allow for one sample, you must sample a sufficient volume of air such that a minimum of 20 particles would be detected if the particle concentration for the largest particle size were at the class limit. If only one sampling location is to be sampled, a minimum of three sample volumes at that location must be taken.

For sample locations greater than 1 and less than 10, the 95% upper confidence level must be calculated and details for this are in Annex B. This Annex also allows for averaging when the number of sample locations is 10 or greater.

The sampling procedure for the DPC in Annex B states that the probe must be positioned directly into the airflow that is being sampled. The interpretations of the results are to assure that the classification requirement has been met. However, if noncompliance is caused by a single nonrandom outlier value with less than 10 sample locations, this value may be called an outlier and this outlier may be excluded from the calculation provided that:

1. The calculation is repeated
2. At least three measurement values remain
3. No more than one measurement is excluded
4. The suspect cause is documented

Of course, the value must be still within the classification level.

ISO 14644-2—Specifications for Testing and Monitoring to Prove Continued Compliance with ISO 14644-1 (7 Pages)

This part of the ISO 14644 series published in 2000 specifies requirements for periodic testing of a cleanroom or clean zone to prove continued compliance with ISO 14644-1 for the designated classification of airborne particulate cleanliness. The common term of "recertification" has been replaced by "requalification," which is defined as the execution of a test sequence specified for the installation to demonstrate compliance with ISO 14644-1 according to the classification of the installation including the verification of selected pretest conditions. The type of routine monitoring for particulates will dictate the maximum time interval between requalifications. As an example, classifications of cleanrooms lower than or equal to ISO Class 5 have a maximum time interval of six months. ISO classifications greater than ISO Class 5 will have a maximum time interval of 12 months.

TABLE 4 Schedule of Testing to Demonstrate Compliance

Test parameter	Maximum time interval (months)	Test procedure
Class of air cleanliness		
≤ ISO Class 5	6	Annex B in ISO 14644-1:1999
> ISO Class 5	12	Annex B in ISO 14644-1:1999
Airflow volume or velocity	12	ISO 14644-3:2005, clause B.4
Air pressure difference	12	ISO 14644-3:2005, clause B.5

However, where the installation is equipped with instrumentation for continuous or frequent monitoring of airborne particle concentration and air pressure differential, the time factor may be extended provided the results of continuous or frequent monitoring remain within the specified limits. Continuous monitoring is defined as updating that occurs constantly. Frequent monitoring is updating that occurs at specified intervals not to exceed 60 minutes during operations. Air flow volume or velocity and air pressure differential are also required tests for requalification. The maximum time interval for these is 12 months (Table 4).

In addition to the normative tests, there are also some optional tests that are indicated in Annex A and these include installed filter leakage, airflow visualization, recovery, and containment leakage.

ISO 14644-3 Test Methods (62 Pages)
This standard published in 2005 specifies the test methods for characterizing the performance of cleanrooms and clean zones. ISO 14644-3 places emphasis on the 13 recommended tests used to characterize cleanrooms and clean zones:

1. Airborne particle count for classification
2. Airborne particle count for ultrafine particles
3. Airborne particle count for macroparticles
4. Airflow
5. Air pressure difference
6. Installed filter system leakage
7. Airflow direction and visualization
8. Temperature
9. Humidity
10. Electrostatic and ion generator
11. Particle deposition
12. Recovery
13. Containment leakage

As identified in ISO 14644-1 and ISO 14644-2, some of these tests are mandatory but most are voluntary. The key controlling factor in the quality level of any cleanroom is the owner's requirements and what measurements are necessary to achieve that level of performance. The overall emphasis of these tests is performance. ISO 14644-3 does not specifically address measurements on product or processes in cleanrooms. Rather, it covers the cleanroom performance characteristics that lead to the ability to measure product and process quality levels as desired by the owner.

Of the 13 recommended cleanroom qualification tests, the choice of which tests are to be applied to a particular cleanroom is per agreement between the buyer and seller. There are three major annexes in this ISO standard.

Annex A is by far the most user friendly as it lists all the recommended tests and provides a means of defining the sequence in which the tests are to be utilized in classifying and qualifying a cleanroom or clean zone.

Annex B details the individual test methods so there can be no misunderstanding between the customer and the supplier, i.e., buyer and seller. Over 60% of the pages of ISO 14644-3 are contained in Annex B. Each test method is carefully described. How the test it to be conducted, any test limitations, and how the test data is reported are presented in this standard.

Annex C of ISO 14644-3 lists the instrumentation that will be used by the 13 recommended tests. The performance parameters for each instrument are given, including the sensitivity limits, measuring range, acceptable error, response time, calibration interval, counting efficiency, and data display. For example, particle counting can be accomplished by utilizing a DPC, a condensation nucleus counter, a cascade impactor, a time of flight particle instrument, or a piezobalance impactor.

It is important to have clearly defined test methods and metrology when the significant investment value of a cleanroom project must rest on very specific referee performance criteria. ISO 14644-3 provides these referee test methods, thereby providing stability and global uniformity to the base performance criteria for world-class cleanrooms and clean zones.

ISO 14644-4—Design, Construction, and Startup (51 Pages)

This part of ISO 14644 published in 2001 specifies the requirements for the design and construction of a cleanroom installation but does not prescribe specific technological or contractual means to meet these requirements. Construction guidance is provided, including the requirements for startup and qualification. Basic elements of design and construction needed to insure continued satisfactory operation are identified through the consideration of relevant aspects of operation and maintenance.

This ISO standard details items that will be needed for planning and design, construction and startup, testing and approval, and documentation. Eight annexes are included in this document.

These annexes describe in detail the basic concepts for designing clean space. For example, what is this space to be used for, what is the proper layout for equipment and personnel access, what type of contamination and choice of construction materials must be considered, how do you handle the environmental parameters, and what is the airflow pattern?

Annex H provides an excellent checklist to assist the user in communicating with the designer on the requirements for the process, equipment, external factors, systems, and other issues that influence the cost, scheduling, and basic design of a cleanroom and other controlled environments. A careful following of the guidance terms spelled out in Annex H is a must for anyone designing, building, or operating clean space.

ISO 14644-5 Operations (44 Pages)

This standard published in 2004 specifies the basic requirements for operating a cleanroom. The standard is divided into six important key elements:

- Operational systems
- Cleanroom clothing
- Personnel

- Stationary equipment
- Materials and portable equipment
- Cleanroom cleaning.

The operational system requirements address the procedures, protocols, and risk factors used to identify the various contamination concerns. System requirements, including documentation and training, are also covered.

The second section discusses cleanroom clothing. The elements include the fabric, laundry, frequency of change, packaging of garments, garment inspection, and other special considerations such as electrostatic discharge, chemical, and microbial fabric concerns and issues.

The third section on personnel addresses storage of personal items, jewelry, and cosmetics, as well as personnel training, behavior, and hygiene.

Stationary equipment must include the installation, maintenance, and preventive maintenance of such equipment. Discussion on cleaning and decontamination of the equipment, as well as admittance to its location for usage, is included.

Materials and portable equipment speak to the appropriate level of cleanliness in reference to the process and products. Proper entry procedures and protocols for bringing items into the cleanroom and removing items such as finished product and waste items from the cleanroom are covered here.

The section on cleanroom cleaning is extensive. This section specifies the methods and procedures, training, schedules, and contamination checks used to ensure that cleanliness has been achieved and the cleanroom controlled environment is maintained at the level for which it was designed.

The six annexes to this ISO standard expound on the normative section in great detail and list actual procedures and examples for each one of these sections. Included in the annexes are a gowning procedure, specific information on training, equipment repair procedures, and detailed cleaning procedures.

ISO 14644-6—Vocabulary (21 Pages)

The scope of this standard to be published in 2007 is to define those terms that require more specific description than is found in normal dictionary sources. ISO 14644-6 is the repository of all of the common terms and definitions used in all the other ISO 14644 and ISO 14698 documents pertaining to cleanrooms and associated controlled environments. It is an alphabetical database of terms applicable to this new family of ISO cleanroom standards. These definitions have been harmonized to allow for uniformity of meaning across these new cleanroom standards.

ISO 14644-7—Separative Devices (Clean Air Hoods, Glove Boxes, Isolators, and Mini Environments) (52 Pages)

This standard published in 2004 covers clean areas that are usually stand-alone and self-sufficient by design. Their other primary criterion is that they are not designed for internal occupancy by personnel, i.e., they are people-free enclosures.

Interestingly, most of the new science in this family of ISO cleanroom standards is in this particular document.

Picture if you will all the information in the other nine cleanroom standards having to be placed into the confined spaces of a smaller controlled clean environment. This is what is classified as a separative device. Examples are clean benches, isolators, glove boxes, and mini environments.

They usually enclose a small research or manufacturing process that not only protects this process from the personnel directly involved but also protects these personnel from the process.

In addition to the confined controlled environment space, there are specific criteria for access devices, transfer devices, leak testing, and special air- and gas-handling systems.

There is a very effective Annex A, which provides a separation continuum concept along with a representative table of eight separation continuum devices defined in general terms. This provides an excellent guidance for determining design, construction, and operational requirements.

ISO 14644-8—Classification of Airborne Molecular Contamination (22 Pages)

This particular standard published in 2006 establishes a rating system for determining airborne molecular contamination in cleanrooms. It provides a system to classify the type of contaminant, the amount of contaminant, and the methods by which it was collected and analyzed. The contaminant categories are acid, base, biotoxic, condensable, corrosive, dopant, organic, oxidant, and specific individual substances where appropriate.

Sources of molecular contamination are described, such as outdoor air, construction materials, process chemicals, process tooling, and personnel. Four typical collection methods are cited along with eight sampling methods.

There are 17 offline analytical methods cited along with 9 online methods. There is a wide variety of choice of collection and analysis to determine the amount and type of airborne molecular contamination. All of this information is then placed into a classification system as follows:

ISO-AMC Class $N(x)$

N is the ISO-AMC class, which is the logarithmic concentration, expressed in g/m^3 within a range of 0 to 12. $N = \log_{10}[\text{concentration in } g/m^3]$; x is the contaminate category.

For example, ISO-AMC Class-6 (NH_3) expresses an airborne concentration of $10^{-6}\,g/m^3$ of ammonia. 10^{-6} is 1 $\mu g/m^3$ or 1000 ng/m^3. These ISO-AMC classes are listed in Table 5.

Annex D of this document provides the specific requirements for measuring and classifying airborne molecular contamination in Separative Devices (ISO 14644-7).

With this knowledge of concentration, cleanroom operators can make value judgments on levels of airborne molecular contamination that is or is not acceptable for quality purposes. A baseline quality level can be established and utilized as an on-going monitoring tool. Anyone concerned with airborne molecular contamination should be using ISO 14644-8 as a baseline quality standard. A companion document on surface molecular contamination is in development and should be published by 2008.

ISO 14698-1 (32 Pages) and ISO 14698-2 (11 Pages) Biocontamination Control

ISO-14698-1 published in 2003 describes the principles and the basic metrology for a formal system to assess and control biocontamination in cleanrooms.

TABLE 5 ISO-AMC Classes

ISO-AMC class	Concentration (g/m^3)	Concentration (μg/m)^3	Concentration (ng/m^3)
0	10^0	10^6 (1,000,000)	10^9 (1,000,000,000)
−1	10^{-1}	10^5 (100,000)	10^8 (100,000,000)
−2	10^{-2}	10^4 (10,000)	10^7 (10,000,000)
−3	10^{-3}	10^3 (1000)	10^6 (1,000,000)
−4	10^{-4}	10^2 (100)	10^5 (100,000)
−5	10^{-5}	10^1 (10)	10^4 (10,000)
−6	10^{-6}	10^0 (1)	10^3 (1000)
−7	10^{-7}	10^{-1} (0.1)	10^2 (100)
−8	10^{-8}	10^{-2} (0.01)	10^1 (10)
−9	10^{-9}	10^{-3} (0.001)	10^0 (1)
−10	10^{-10}	10^{-4} (0.0001)	10^{-1} (0.1)
−11	10^{-11}	10^{-5} (0.00001)	10^{-2} (0.01)
−12	10^{-12}	10^{-6} (0.000001)	10^{-3} (0.001)

As international trade in hygiene-sensitive products increases, there is a strong requirement for stable and safe products, particularly in the health-care field. Achieving this stability and safety requires the control of biocontamination in the design, specifications, operation, and controls of cleanrooms and associated controlled environments.

ISO 14698-1 provides guidance principles for establishing and maintaining a formal system to assess biocontamination controls in these special environments. It is important to have a formal system that can assess and control factors that will affect the microbiological quality of a product or process. There are a number of formalized systems to achieve this, such as hazard analysis critical control points, fault tree analysis, failure mode and effect analysis, and others. ISO 14698-1 is concerned only with a formal system to address microbiological hazards in cleanrooms. Such a system must have the means of identifying the potential hazard, determine the resilient likelihood of occurrence, designate risk zones, establish measures of prevention or control, establish control limits, establish monitoring and observation schedules, establish corrective action, establish training programs, and provide proper documentation. It is the user's responsibility to develop, initiate, implement, and document a formal system for biocontamination control—one that enables detection of adverse conditions in a timely fashion. Certain regulatory authorities will have significant impact on this responsibility. Target, alert, and action levels must be determined for any given risk zone. Such levels will determine the required remediation effect. All these factors impact product quality.

A biocontamination sampling program must be established for cleanroom air, walls, floors, ceilings, process equipment, raw materials, processed liquids and gases, furniture, storage containers, personnel attire, and protective clothing. Sampling frequency site locations, sample identification, culturing methods, and evaluation criteria must be included. This formal system becomes a key part of the validation process for a cleanroom or associated controlled environment.

ISO 14698-1 also provides detailed guidance on how to measure airborne biocontamination, how to validate air samplers, and how to measure biocontamination of surfaces, liquids, and textiles used in cleanrooms. It also provides guidance for validating laundry processes and how to provide proper personnel training. ISO 14698-1 has a companion document ISO 14698-2, which provides guidance on the evaluation and interpretation of biocontamination data.

The scope of ISO 14698-2 published in 2003 gives guidance on basic principles and metrology requirements of all microbiological data evaluation obtained from sampling for viable particles in specified risk zones in cleanrooms. Determining the presence and significance of biocontamination is a multistep task. Sampling techniques, time factors, culturing techniques, and analysis methods (qualitative or quantitative) have to be carefully planned. Target, alert, and action levels have to be determined for each risk zone based on the initial biocontamination data, collection, and evaluation plan. Each enumeration technique must be validated, considering the viable particles involved. Good data and evaluation documentation is necessary to determine trend analysis and the quality of risk zones. All the specification results require verification. ISO 14698-2 provides the guidance for answering all these concerns.

SUMMARY

The 10 ISO documents outlined above represent Phase One of the work if ISO/TC 209. They provide a strong baseline of ISO standards for cleanrooms and associated controlled environments used in the research and manufacture of quality products. This is particularly applicable to those products that cannot be adequately manufactured in a nonclean environment.

These 10 ISO documents are living standards. By ISO rules, they have to be reviewed every five years. All ISO nations are asked to review each document, offer comments, and indicate the continuing use of the document. Comments received are given to ISO/TC 209 for acceptance or rejection and the particular standards is either left as is, modified, or terminated as appropriate.

This five-year review process is part of Phase Two of the work of ISO/TC 209. In addition, new work has been started on surface particulate contamination and surface molecular contamination to establish methods of measurement, analysis, and classification.

Phase Two also allows for ISO/TC 209 to stay abreast of changing cleanroom technology and industry needs. ISO/TC 209 now has formal liaison with the newly formed ISO/TC 229 on nanotechnology. The future of expanding needs for cleanrooms and associated controlled environments is upon us.

Copies of the ISO 14644 and ISO 14698 standards can be obtained from the Institute of Environmental Sciences and Technology (1).

REFERENCE

1. www.IEST.org.

3 Cleanroom Certification and Particulate Testing

David Brande

- Introduction
- High-Efficiency Particulate Air Filters
- Pharmaceutical Introduction
- Air Volumes
- Practical Application
- Airflow Patterns
- Practical Application
- Pressure
- Filter Integrity
- Practical Application
- Bleedthrough
- Room Classification
- Practical Application
- Conclusion

Cleanroom Certification and Particulate Testing

David Brande

NNE-US, Inc., Clayton, North Carolina, U.S.A.

INTRODUCTION

To begin, let us get a clear definition of what we will be discussing in this chapter—do you have a "clean room," or do you have a "cleanroom?" Of course as we know from growing up, when it is separated into two different words—clean and room—that is what your mother always wanted to have. As one word, it lays the foundation of our current desire for a controlled environment in which we are trying to minimize detriment caused by particulate, either viable or nonviable.

In this chapter, we are going to discuss cleanroom certification in the pharmaceutical, bio-pharma, and Medical Device industry as an Food and Drug Administration (FDA)-regulated controlled environment and to the practicality of providing that service in the context of current requirements and procedures both nationally and internationally.

Now by definition, and this is out of IEST-RP-CC006.3, a cleanroom is "a room in which the air supply, air distribution, filtration of the air supply, materials of construction, and operating procedures are regulated to control particle concentration so that an appropriate air cleanliness class, as defined in ISO14644-1, 1999 can be met."

HIGH-EFFICIENCY PARTICULATE AIR FILTERS

When talking about certifying the effectiveness of controlled environment areas, consider the membrane that actually creates this environment that we desire for the production of our quality products. That membrane is what we refer to as high-efficiency particulate air (HEPA) filtration. The standard filter that is most common is a 2-ft. by 4-ft. (2×4) ceiling-mounted filter that filters the incoming supply air. These filters are supplied by a large number of manufacturers worldwide, some have been around for 50 years or more, and others are newer to the industry, but the supply of filters is very prominent within the industry.

We cannot talk about HEPA filters without first understanding a little bit about their history which goes all the way back to the World War I gas and chemical warfare. Of course, the urgency of the moment was to try to guard against long-term damage or even death of the individuals fighting in the war. It was not until World War II that we discovered that a mixture of asbestos and cellulose combined would make quite a good filtering device. This discovery came with the capture of a German gas mask in which the filtering mechanism was from a company by the name of Drager. Of course, the information was top secret throughout World War II and as part of our American history, the "new" filter technology was used in what is now known as the top secret research of the Manhattan project. The work that was being done on the development of the nuclear bomb resulted in a need for a level of filtration that only a HEPA filter could provide. Later the governmental group known as the Manhattan project morphed into the Atomic

Energy Commission of the United States and today HEPA filters are a prominent fixture in nuclear containment.

That early association with the U.S. military, resulted in what we refer to as Military Specifications (MIL-SPECS) associated with a type media that we use known as MIL-SPEC F-15079B and then of course, the MIL-SPEC for testing of filter media is 282. Even after World War II, these MIL-SPECS were still classified and only the U.S. government used them, but in the 1950s that information was declassified and four companies began producing HEPA filters for the government and subsequently for general consumption.

It was this beginning that set up the use almost immediately of what we now refer to as microelectronics industry's need for the use of HEPA filters. The military was already using the filters for the assembly of mechanical devices that were utilized in missiles and airplanes. As things became more and more miniaturized and dust particles were more and more critical, of course, it was just natural that microelectronics was the first to start utilizing HEPA filters in a production environment.

What I would like to do now is go back and talk briefly about each of the tests needed to qualify a cleanroom and some of the problems that you will run into trying to actually perform the tests and considerations that need to be taken into account in reporting the data.

PHARMACEUTICAL INTRODUCTION

It was after microelectronics that pharmaceutical began using the HEPA filters for primary supply filtration and then shortly followed by medical device and then food processing. Of course, other industries that are coming along such as the automobile painting industry are using HEPA filters also. Even so, all have roots in the Atomic Energy Commission from World War II.

The HEPA filter utilizes three collection mechanisms of physics that allow them to collect most of the particulate matter, hence their original nomenclature of the "absolute filter." Those mechanisms are impaction, interception, and diffusion. There are other mechanisms, but these are the primary forces of our HEPA filter. In the beginning, we were interested in a particle size of one-half micron (0.50 μm), the smallest that could be measured with some degree of confidence and this particle size became the basis for the English-based cleanroom classification system. Therefore, Class 100 (or Class 10,000) meant there could be as many as 100 (or 10,000) half-micron particles per cubic foot of air.

We will address this more later on in this chapter as we speak directly about room classification. To give you kind of a context of what the particle sizes we seek to collect with the HEPA filter, the average human hair is about 100 microns wide; therefore, something that is one-half of a micron is roughly one-200th of the width of a human hair.

Of course, the overall efficiency is what we are interested in when we talk about these filters and 0.3 μm became the particle size that we thought was going to be the most difficult to capture. We are talking about research that was done through the 1950s and 1960s and so most of the American standards still refer to efficiency ratings at 0.3 μm with dioctyl phthalate (DOP). This was actually a theoretical calculation and with the advance of both science and equipment, we have since determined that 0.3 μm is not the most difficult particle size to collect, but rather a particle size somewhat smaller. Therefore, 0.3 μm is not necessarily the best measurement for the true efficiency of a filter, something to be covered later.

At this point, let us talk about why we would want to certify a cleanroom, after all the filters are tested at the factory. First, we have got to verify conformance with the design and the procurement specifications. In other words, have we gotten what we paid for? Also, you have to check for proper handling and installation, validate that the filtration's system's performance is what was required, and make sure that compliance with any regulatory pressures, say from the FDA. Then, of course, we need to satisfy any kind of quality control or yield issues or meet any International Standards Organization (ISO) requirements that we are working with.

What are the minimal requirements? The specific standard you are using is going to have anywhere from 13 to 15 different tests that are being offered for testing different parameters of the cleanroom's performance. Many of these tests are industry-specific; in other words, not everyone is interested in accomplishing the end result of say a vibration test, something very critical to microelectronics or Medical Device industries but not so critical to the bio-pharma industry. The same applies to tests like, say room-parallelism, meaning that the air is remains parallel while moving through the room. Again, critical in microelectronics not so critical in bio-pharma or Medical Device industries because the rooms are primarily designed with side wall returns.

So I propose to you if a room can be shown to successfully provide four different methods of particulate control, then the room is certified. This qualification will require four tests under normal conditions. If you have an ISO 5 or cleaner, then we have one additional test that we would recommend. I would like to discuss what it is that we are trying to prove when we perform these four tests.

First Postulate:
Show that if particulate does enter the controlled environment, the particulate will be disposed of in a timely and efficient manner.

For the higher classifications, we utilize room air exchange rates, the result of measuring the volume of air provided to the room and then taking into account the cubic volume of the room. Then if certifying an ISO 5 or cleaner, there will be a need for airflow visualization to demonstrate exactly what is happening with the air flow through the room.

AIR VOLUMES

Now when it comes to measuring the room air exchange rates and documenting the airflow visualization, the tests are fairly easily done. You are going to determine the actual supply volume coming into the room and there may be some uniformity requirements. Some clients like to have uniformity between the filters, if there are multiple filters in a room. And then, of course, you add all of those supplies to get a total volume of the room. I recommend that these measurements be made with a flow hood (Fig. 1) when possible, which collects all of the air exiting from a filter and sends it through a fixed measuring device, called a tube array. The measuring of all of the air volume is more accurate than any other method.

When you cannot use a hood, most of the manufacturers who have the electronic micromanometers also have what they call a tube array (Fig. 2) that can be

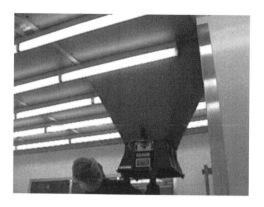

FIGURE 1 Proper application of a flow hood to determine filter volume.

utilized to read velocity pressure directly on the filter face, which then automatically converted to velocity, which can later be converted to volume manually. Ultimately, volume is what we want to have.

Next on the list is using a thermal anemometer (Fig. 3) to read velocity. Whenever you use any device other than the flow hood device, you will lose some level of accuracy and consistency in being able to depict what is the true volume of the filter.

Finally, a device that was once popular and is again having some resurgence into popularity is the vane anemometer. The vane anemometer (Fig. 4) helps to dampen some of the fluctuations both in direction and speed that are taking place in the filters, as a result of the newly designed filters we now have in the marketplace with a high degree of variation in filter face velocity.

Once you collect all the volumes, either by direct measurement or conversion, simply divide it into the room volume and multiply it by 60 and you will have what your room air exchange rates are per hour.

$$\frac{\text{Room volume}}{\text{Supply volume}} \times 60 = \text{air changes} / \text{hour}$$

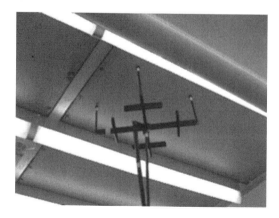

FIGURE 2 Proper use of tube array to determine filter face velocity.

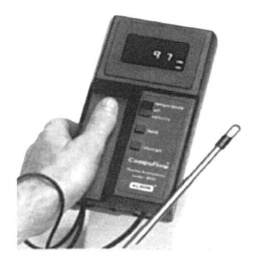

FIGURE 3 Example of hot wire anemometer.

    With the multiple documents in the industry now, none agree on what the maximum and minimum rates should be at each desired level of cleanliness, but we do have some overlap. Generally, each level will contain the desired rates that have been shared through government guidelines or the like. For example, each recommended list will include 20 air changes per hour (a minimum established by the FDA in the aseptic guidelines) in the range of the lowest level of a controlled environment.

PRACTICAL APPLICATION

As mentioned before, volumetric measurements are what we are looking for. Using the flow hood attached to a permanently affixed grid in which the micromanometer reads the difference between total pressure and static pressure, which in turn can yield velocity pressure that can be converted to velocity. Knowing the area that the grid is fixed, you can easily make a conversion to a volumetric measurement. This is desirable because you are reading the entire volume of air that is being distributed by the filter delivery system. In my experience, if five technicians

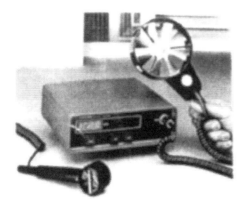

FIGURE 4 Example of a vane anemometer.

read the same filter, they are going to come back with numbers that are very close to each other resulting in the desirability of measuring volumetrically.

When you need to read in velocities, the tube array would be desired as part of the micromanometer set. Again if five people to make the same measurement, the variation is going to be a little bit wider because of how each one places the tube array on the filter screen or how many readings they take as the others that measured the velocities. Introduce more variability; get greater variability in the results!

With an anemometer, the variability extrapolates itself even greater because you are only measuring a very small area of the filter. You may take eight readings in which all eight readings accumulatively represent less than 2 in. of filter face, due to the size of the probe inlet. But then we are going to multiply that to be representative of the almost 1000 in.^{2} that a 2×4 filter face makes up, if there is an error or if there is variability, once you extrapolate it to such large numbers, it becomes a significant number that needs to be taken into account.

Whereas reading volumes, there is a better understanding of exactly what is being delivered. There is no better way to sample a population (measure the volume of air) than to measure the entire population, without statistically sampling (as in velocities).

When determining the room air exchange rates, normally the user is looking for an even threshold number like a minimum of 20 air changes or a minimum of 60 air changes. So when making measurements of the room, do not take into account any fixtures if the room air exchange rates are not close to being at their threshold.

For example, in looking for a minimum of 20 taking into account width, length, and height of the room, you have 27 air changes per hour. You are not interested in whether that there is cabinetry in the room. On the other hand, if a room measured at say 19 air changes per hour, then you may want to go in and take out the volume that a permanent tank or any other permanent fixtures such as cabinetry or pylons that actually take up volume of the room. By taking those into account, you get a truer reading of room air exchange rates.

AIRFLOW PATTERNS

In an ISO 5 cleanroom, after the room air exchange rates are established, the user may require some form of airflow visualization, sometimes referred to as "smoke pattern testing" or "airflow pattern testing." Airflow visualization is a more descriptive test. "Smoke" infers a more destructive test than it actually is and the reference to "pattern" clearly indicates a condition that is not always present. Airflow visualization has become very popular primarily because of its definitive characterization in that the test truly "shows" what is happening inside a room and the visualization will lead to a lot of understanding of what is happening in terms of particulate control and of course how the process equipment can affect the flow of air through the work area.

PRACTICAL APPLICATION

This test is highly subjective; as a result, a lot of people have different ideas about how to produce it. The aerosol used must be physically capable of showing you what is happening with the airflow movement. For example, a carbon-dioxide-generated plume using dry ice is extremely colder than the surrounding ambient air. Naturally, the plume will drop just like the cold air that falls into the room once a freezer door is opened. You will have the same effect if you try and use this in a traditional controlled environment. Also, an additional drawback to dry ice is the short plume created that proves to be difficult to capture on film past a couple of feet.

Many certifiers, including myself, have had good results using a theatrical fog generator that has a mixture of glycol. However, this fluid does leave a residue that may require a cleaning validation and product and equipment compatibility testing. After the airflow visualization test using an appropriate aerosol, cleaning is recommended. In situations where aseptic cleanliness was paramount, an alternative is a hydrosonic humidifiers supplied with water for injection. However, this type of generated plume is very difficult to videotape unlike the theatrical fog, which has a very long trail. A *major* drawback in using theatrical fog is that it *will* set off a fire alarm system, so you do need to be aware that the fire alarms need to be shut down, with permission of the safety department and the local fire Marshall.

You can do an individual plume as simple as an individual holding the generator and holding the delivery tube as they walk through an area. By modifying a delivery system, with several holes, multiple plumes will allow you to cover 3, 4, 6, 8 ft. at one time. The method utilized should always provide the user with documented results in VHS videotape or DVD of your cleanroom or process. One of the things that may be very useful is an Apple program called iMovie and iDVD (there are comparable programs for the PC). In the field, a white board can be used for filming and specific clip information. This documentation will assist the user in the compilation of the video.

Second Postulate:
The second postulate was that we must demonstrate that no particulate will enter the controlled environment as a result of construction. Of course, we do that by performing room pressure differential.

PRESSURE

We can qualify through pressure differentials the ability to keep particulate either in or out depending on what is required. Room pressurization as a test is probably the simplest and easiest of the tests to accomplish in the sense that it is literally the difference in pressure across a doorway between two different rooms and more importantly two different classifications.

A production area can be either positive or negative depending on what is being produced. If you are producing a vaccine, you most likely have the room under negative pressure and if you are producing insulin or a Medical device, you have it under positive pressure. Yet you have all these inlets and outlets and doorways and mouse holes for the product to migrate through. We can measure through pressure differentials the ability to keep particulate either in or out depending on the desire. Remember that the first requirement is to verify the capability that the production area can maintain specified a room pressure differential between the cleanroom and the surrounding areas.

Pressure differentials can be measured by a variety of different pieces of equipment. Also, ideally you need to do this test after the completion of the airflow-related tests such as airflow volume and velocities. Before measuring pressures, you need to make sure that the room is operating at its proper airflows and any adjustments have been made.

The most popular piece of equipment is the modern day electronic micromanometer. You can also use the traditional incline manometer, which has been used for years and even a mechanical differential pressure gage can be utilized to read pressures. The equipment is easy to utilize and easy to set up. Measurements in the United States are predominantly done in inches of water gage, but we are seeing more and more of the requirement for measurements in pascals, which is the European measurement that can convert to millimeters instead of inches.

The FDA has given us guidelines, starting in 1987, stating that they would like for this pressure to be 0.05 in. of water gage. Currently, the FDA has clarified that goal in the current guidelines of September 2004 in that the pressure differential between classes needs to be 0.05 in. of water gage. Sometimes within an area of production, you will have similar rooms operating and often times those pressures will be less than 0.05, but you need to remember that if there is a classification change, we need to make sure that it is 0.05. If you are within a classification, you need to have the cleanest area more positive than the less clean (or the reverse if your goal is to maintain negative pressure) and the most positive area to be the center of what they refer to as the pressure bulls eye with pressures cascading outward. So if you have a similar area, say of ISO 5, you need to have at least a 0.03 and often companies use air locks to achieve these pressure differentials between areas inside the same classification.

Third postulate:
You need to establish that no particulate can enter the controlled environment through the supply air system.

In order to prove this, you will need to perform the in-place integrity test and to do that you would utilize photometers and an oil aerosol such as polyalpha olefin (PAO). Photometers along with an oil aerosol will yield the best test results as to the integrity of the installed filers.

FILTER INTEGRITY

Integrity testing is the most physical and the most difficult to perform of all the tests recommended. Just the sheer task of scanning every square inch of filter face for integrity and document any bypass of the system itself is very labor-intensive. The difficulty in acquiring a significant upstream challenge to the system to ensure that the test is valid can also prove difficult. This is one of the several reasons why the FDA has insisted in the past on using an oil-based aerosol challenge to secure the integrity of the filters. If you start deviating from a photometric measured oil-based aerosol challenge, you add additional factors that can effect the reported outcome and the validity of the work.

First, why would you want to test a HEPA filter once onsite and installed (in situ) when they have already been tested and certified by the factory of the manufacturer? There are actually many reasons for testing after installation. First, and probably most important, the factory actually grades the filter with an efficiency test. The simplest definition of an efficiency test would be to measure the particulate upstream of the filter and then measure the particulate downstream of the filter, that fractional component of those two numbers gives us the overall efficiency of the filter in percent, such as 99.97% efficient at collecting 0.3 μm particles.

From the more practical side, there can be shipping damage as a result of just the physical movement of the filters in trucks across the country also the removal of those filters by inexperienced people from the trucks to the loading docks and then on into the production areas for installation, by either trained or untrained installation personnel and also whether they were properly installed into the filter housings. Many new construction areas hire individuals installing the filters had never seen HEPA filters before given the task of instillation, needless to say, a recipe for a potentially undesirable outcome. Remember that the HEPA filter is only one component of the entire system that is used to establish particulate control over the production area.

Let me return to the grading system for a moment, which can be very critical in understanding the purchase of the correct filter for the application at hand. Over the years, industry has added different grades of filters because applications have changed in both use and advancement in technology. For a long period, only grade levels of A, B, C, D, E, and F. The first three, A, B, and C, were both MIL-STD manufactured and tested. (Institute of Environmental Sciences—IEST RP-001.) These grades of filters were primarily used in the pharmaceutical industry, in particular, C, due to the two additional test methods associated with the classification before the filter left the factory. To explain the classification further, a grade A filter meant that the filter has been tested with an oil aerosol at rated flow. A grade B filter meant that the filter is also tested at 20% of rated flow, with an oil aerosol. A grade C filter meant that the filter has then been hand-scanned by an individual, sometimes by robotics, with a form of oil aerosol that is used in the field. Why is this so important? You can have a hole in a filter and pass total penetration but the requirement in the bio/pharmaceutical industry is no filter with holes and no leaks greater than 0.01%. For this reason, C filters are very popular in bio-pharma, because the factory testing of scanning the filter is very similar to what will be done on site after installation.

The filter grade F, originally intended primarily for microelectronics, was the first deviation from MIL-SPEC and came about after we discovered more about the actual efficiency of the filters in terms of something smaller of 0.3 microns was the most difficult to collect. These filters are ultra-low particulate air (ULPA) filters.

All these filter grades can be found in the Institute of Environmental Sciences and Technologies (IEST), recommended practice (RP), for contamination control (CC001) currently at revision 1.4. The newest revision has included more filter grades to the sequence and now has grades G, H, I, J, and K added. Remember that filter grades A, B, and C are produced and tested to MIL-SPEC standards, whereas the grade F filter production and test requirements come from another recommended practice, IEST RP CC007 ULPA filters.

PRACTICAL APPLICATION

Now let us discuss these individual tests and how we would perform them in the field different from the factory. Aerosol generation, hot DOP versus cold DOP, pretty much sums up the difference between the factory testing and what is done in the field. Hot DOP is an MIL-SPEC requirement involving a large and expensive piece of equipment in the factory that can create a monodisbursed aerosol of 0.3 μm which what we historically wanted to test at, thinking that that was the most

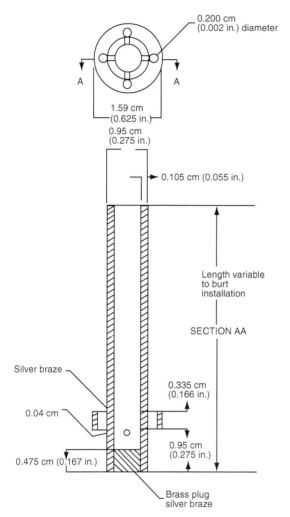

FIGURE 5 Design specifications for a Laskin nozzle.

difficult particle to collect. In the field, cold DOP generation of a polydispersed oil aerosol is used because that is what technology has provided.

We can generate a cold oil aerosol through the use of Laskin nozzles (Fig. 5) for small pieces of equipment up to a few thousand cubic feet per minute (cfm). When the requirement is for larger pieces of equipment, i.e., air handlers up to about 50,000 cfm, thermal generators are used. Thermal generators (Fig. 6) are often confused with hot DOP generation but they are only hot in the sense that the equipment operates at high temperature (760°F) but the distribution of the aerosol is still considered polydisbursed and currently a little bit smaller than 0.3 µm. So the factory is set up to test the filters C type much like we test them in the field with a polydisbursed aerosol and using Laskin nozzles. In field testing, an in-place integrity test requires a full media scan (Fig. 7). It also includes the joints, the frames, the ceiling itself in which the filter housing has been place. Of course, the gaskets and any other seals that may be associated with separating that

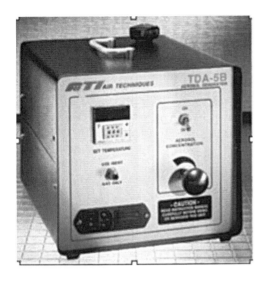

FIGURE 6 An example of a thermal generator.

room from the outside environment. To do that, we have to be prepared to run a successful challenge, in the field, with enough aerosol upstream that we can be confident that the filters are leak-free.

In the past, one customer had an area where discrete particle counters had been used to scan the HEPA filters in a production facility for seven years. After testing with photometers and oil aerosol, it was determined that the filters were riddled with leaks and some as big as 80% with light fixtures that leaked greater than 20%. Remember that any leak greater than 0.01% needs to be repaired. It was obvious that these large leaks had been overlooked or missed on prior certifications, supporting the fact that the scanning method was improperly applied. The point that I want to make is that is not the test method (integrity testing using discrete particle counters) that is not good, but rather it is a very difficult and very complex for untrained people to utilize and perform in the field, for a multitude of reasons. Normally discrete particle counter scanning has to be performed at a much slower rate than the traditional oil-based aerosol with photometry. Again, the differences between these two tests are something that you need to keep in mind when ordering one over the other test.

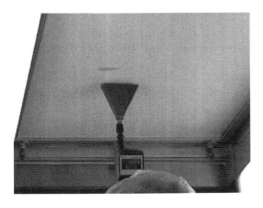

FIGURE 7 Proper scanning of a HEPA filter with a photometer.

BLEEDTHROUGH

Currently in the industry, there has been a shift in the manufacture of high-efficiency filters and no longer is the heavy grade MIL-SPEC filters (99.99% efficient at 0.3 μm) readily available. Again, this is why we now have filter grades A to K to allow for this large variation in how filters can be made.

If you order an old-style filter, 99.99% efficient at 0.3 μm, the filter will in fact be efficient at that level, but for any particulate smaller than 0.3 μm, efficiency could drop off quickly for that filter. Regarding the test methodology that we have been using for the past 40 years, we have recently discovered that we have been testing filters in the field at a particle smaller than 0.3 μm, more or less in the 0.25–0.27 μm size. The result is significant mass leakage through the filter media into the production area and this is a phenomenon that has been around for since the early 1990s called bleedthrough. Everyone needs to be aware when ordering filters especially in a pharmaceutical application where you are currently restricted to the test methodology of oil-based aerosol with photometric test equipment, that we are going to end up testing with this smaller particle and you must understand that this is not the equivalent filter that we were using say ten or twelve years ago, when your facility was built. So in the process of reordering, you should consider this issue of bleedthrough most likely. When reordering and told "that filter designation has been changed to ..." beware! You will have bleedthrough.

With a Laskin nozzle generator, you will not have the bleedthrough issue. This phenomenon is only associated with thermal generators of all makes and models, those generators that are designed to be utilized in air handlers 3000 to 50,000 cfm. This is addressed in IEST RP CC0034, a RP for testing HEPA and ULPA filters.

Once you have completed the integrity testing of an area, you need to document any leaks that have been found in any of the filters in the area of the production area that you were testing. Some will do this simply by listing the filters by their filter numbers. However, some will go as far as to place a rendering of the filter on paper, where the approximate location of the leak is documented. By doing this in terms of a room or multiple rooms and showing the approximate locations, you are able to reduce the amount of paperwork that you have to handle.

Fourth Postulate:
In conclusion, you must show that the controlled environment can produce and maintain the desired room classification.

From inception, certain rooms were set up to be designated levels of particulate control with room classifications according to the ISO 14644-1 *Air cleanliness classes.* These levels of cleanliness are determined for each room based on an accepted statistical method of collecting particle counts for each classification. Room classification differs dramatically from monitoring in that the former is an issue of design and construction and the latter is related to the production of the final product.

ROOM CLASSIFICATION

When collecting data for the room classification, one of the things that you have got to take into account is that there are three stated levels of activity for a cleanroom that it can be tested at, but in the pharmaceutical applications only two of the three are used. In microelectronics, we have an "as-built" state, which tests just the room, clear of any equipment, and personnel. Bio-pharma does not use this first level of testing because there really no difference between as-built and as-rest in a bio-pharma application because no adjustments can be made to the floor. Medical Device may wish to use the "as-built" state, but it is not mandatory. The next level of activity use is called "at-rest" which means that all the equipment has been installed, but no personnel are present. In some applications, this activity level is often referred to as "static conditions." The final level of classification is "operational" and allows for testing to be performed while both equipment and personnel are present and working. This final stage of testing is often referred to as "dynamic conditions" in some applications.

Federal Standard 209 was the standard for room classification that we utilized for many years, but currently ISO 14644 part 1 is the recognized international standard. To begin a room certification, you first need to establish the number of locations ($N_L = \sqrt{A}$; N_L = Number of locations rounded up to next and A = area in square meters) and then lay out those locations in a grid within the room to give a systematic and representative chance for every area of the room to pass or fail.

If there are less than 10 locations for the area being tested, there are procedures provided for in the ISO standard to do a statistical analysis and create an upper confidence level (UCL) of 95%. When laying out your test grid take into account the room shape and of course the critical process areas that are present in the area.

Remember that you always test a specific particle size when classifying a room. Therefore, an area is classified to a particular size of particle such as an area is ISO Class X at X.X microns and larger (e.g., ISO Class 5 at 0.5 µm and larger or ISO 7 at 5.0 µm and larger).

Let us discuss the actual room classification or the taking of discrete particle counts within an area to classify the particulate level in that area. As I mentioned before, Federal Standard 209 was the first document written to discuss how you would actually take these particle counts to classify an area, and was written in the early 1960s. One of the FS209 versions, FS209B, stayed around a long time, published in the early 1970s, the version was replaced in 1987 with version FS209C. That version quickly became FS209D due to some technical issues and once again, in short order, we ended up with our final version of the standard, which was Federal Standard 209E.

FS209E was both metric and English, in that we still utilized the customary classifications of Class 100, Class 10,000, and Class 100,000 but there were also metric equivalents for those standards and they were listed as SI. For instance, an SI 3.5 was Class 100, 5.5 was Class 10,000, and 6.5 were a Class 100,000. FS209E was very popular and often used throughout the world. With the publishing of the ISO 14644-1, the United States was obligated to sunset the Federal Standard 209 which was successfully done in November 2001. Since the sun setting of Federal Standard, there is only one standard for classification and that is ISO 14644-1, an international standard which lists classified areas from ISO 1 measuring 0.1 size particles through ISO 9 allowing up to 1 million 0.5 particles per cubic foot. From a practical standpoint, even though there is 81 classification levels in the ISO document, in other words a person could be certified to 5.4 or 5.6, bio-pharma does not utilize the in between classifications. Instead, bio-pharma, will use the traditional ISO Classes 5, 6, 7, and 8, which is the English equivalent of Classes 100, 1000, 10,000, and 100,000 in that order.

Even though the new ISO standard is only metric and there is no mention of cubic feet, we still cannot get away from the fact that almost all the particle counters used throughout the world today, still measure in one cubic foot or as they are reported now 28.3 cubic liters per minute. This is still remains the basis of making all of our measurements. We still make our measurements on one cubic foot but now we extrapolate that measurement to quantify a cubic meter. Some manufactures have begun producing what they refer to as "high volume" samplers that sample either at 2 cfm or 50 L/min.

Some users within the United States are still having some difficulty in understanding an ISO 5 versus an ISO 7 area. In the last few years, since the Federal Standard has been sunsetted, often times we will include in our reporting "U.S. customary Class 100" or "U.S. customary Class 10,000" to describe an area that is ISO Class 5 or ISO Class 7 area. Much like the Federal Standard 209B which remained in the nomenclature long after it was replaced, I am quite sure we will still see the nomenclature for stating the number of 0.5 particles allowed per cubic foot will still be utilized into the near future as away to refer to classified areas, but within the ISO standard, it is very explicit about the proper nomenclature

PRACTICAL APPLICATION

One of the big differences in converting from the Federal Standard 209E and the ISO 14644-1 standard is in the statistical analysis of determining locations. In the old Federal Standard, we used to take into account the classification level you were attempting to classify at. For example, to determine the number of sample locations you would first take the square root of the desired classification level to determine the amount of square foot area that each count would represent.

Therefore, in a Class 100,000 area or as we now know an ISO 8, each count would represent $316 \, \text{ft}^2$. Even in a very large room, you only had to take counts at few locations to classify the area. In contrast, if you were testing a critical area, such as Class 100, each count would represent approximately $10 \, \text{ft}^2$ and a lot more counts were needed. With the statistical analysis currently under the ISO, the determination was made there was not the need for that level of stratification. Whether it is an ISO 4 or an ISO 8, the number of count locations is based on the square root of the area in meters to be classified. In other words, it does not matter what the classification level, the number of locations are always going to be the same, if the area remains the same.

So now how does that effect the transition between those of us who have been testing by Federal Standard 209 for all these years trying to transition into the ISO. First, it means that in your critical Class 100 areas, you are going to take less counts than you have been. The Class 1000 and the Class 10,000 not that different, in that the number of locations will still come out within a digit or so of what they were. In the Class 100,000 areas where you have been taking less counts, you are going to end up taking considerably more counts in those areas. You will find this the biggest difference between the old FS209 standard and the new ISO international standard.

The statistical analysis of the data that are collected still remains almost unchanged although there is currently some debate about whether or not the current statistical analysis that we are using currently is sufficient and will be subject of debate. Especially in the upcoming year or so as we are reevaluating the ISO

14644-1 because the standard has reached its five-year anniversary date and therefore is subject to an obligatory reevaluation and restructuring if agreed among the voting nations.

When calculating the number of particle count locations, the square rooting of the room area will always give an number to some decimal point. In both the old and the new standards, a fractional number is automatically raised to the next whole integer. If the calculation results in a number such as 3.89, then you must round up to four locations. And if you come up with 3.01, you are still going to go to four as the number of locations.

The easiest thing to do because most rooms are rectangular or square is to always go for an even number to be evenly spaced within the area. For example, if you had a room that required seven counts and it was either square or rectangular, we would probably go ahead and do eight counts in that area so that we could evenly distribute the locations throughout the room. If the room has an odd shape to it, then it could be accepting of an odd number of counts, if you have a little alcove off to the side that would warrant an additional location. I cannot say it strong enough, when in doubt—always take more locations than you need if there is anything question. If you do not, when you return to the office and do final calculations and find out that the answer was not 3.89 but it was actually 4.03 then you are one location short because you rounded it up to 4, should have been rounded to 5 and you are going to have to go back and take one more count in the area. There is never a penalty for additional counts that are being taken.

When taking the counts, the biggest problem is that the sampling tube is not properly cleaned prior to testing. Even though the technician may run the zero count filter, the tube itself by just sitting in the case or sitting in the truck has accumulated particles in it. Most often, a failure occurs with the first counts of the day, traditionally one of the two situations are the resultant cause. Either when starting up the first location of the day and we are pulling in these large particles and numerous particles that have been lying in the tube or after going from an area of high classification, say an ISO 8 to an ISO 5 area and the tube is loaded up with the particles that have collected on the inner sides of the tube. Therefore, the cleaning of the tubes is definitely a requirement and being aware of that and shaking them because they are going through the zero count filters to make sure that the tube is being cleared of particles. The particle counting probe must always be orientated into the airflow. You can put the zero count filter on your sampling tube and shake the tube and you know that no particles are coming through the zero count filter but you will still register particles that are all coming out of the tubing that is being used for collection. Generally, during certification, only one sample per location is taken.

In terms of the locations, just as with the old Federal Standard and of course with the new ISO 14644-1 statistics, that when you have a minimum number of locations, in other words less than 10, you need to be aware that there is additional UCL that needs to be determined, such as the 95% UCL.

Now if you are only doing one location, you are okay, you just have to three counts in the one location. Of course, it would be an area smaller than $1\,m^2$ to accomplish that. So it would be more like a closet or a small piece of production equipment. Anywhere between two and nine locations, there is a systematic accounting to reach the 95% UCL that will have to be done for each location.

For routine monitoring, the sample locations will be selected by reviewing the certification data and also by performing a risk analysis of the critical points for the process and product. Routine monitoring should combine room as well as process and product locations.

CONCLUSION

These five tests that we have just discussed a little bit are five tests that are centered around the HEPA filtration system itself, the membrane that separates the production area from any uncontrolled environment be it the warehouse or the office area.

There is another series of tests that we refer to as optional and this particular group of optional tests which are airflow parallelism test, the enclosure integrity or induction leak test, the recovery test, and the particle fallout count test are all tests that involve air movement and particle migration. There are five tests, which are both environmental and worker-comfort oriented. Listed they would be lighting level, noise level, temperature, and moisture test and finally vibration testing (Institute of Environmental Sciences—IEST RP 006 and ISO 14644-3—Cleanrooms and Associated Controlled Environments: Test Methods).

4 Monitoring of Airborne Viable Particles

Bengt Ljungqvist and Berit Reinmüller

4 Monitoring of Airborne Viable Particles

Bengt Ljungqvist and Berit Reinmüller
Building Services Engineering, KTH, Stockholm, Sweden

INTRODUCTION

Monitoring of airborne viable particles could be considered as a specific form of aerosol measurement. The term "aerosol" means an assembly of liquid or solid particles in a gaseous medium (e.g., air) stabile enough to enable observation and measurement. Generally, the size of aerosol particles is in the range 0.001 to 100 µm (1).

Particle size, shape, and density determine the behavior of the particle in air. A commonly used term in aerosol science and technology is the aerodynamic diameter, which is the diameter of a unit-density sphere (1 g/cm³) having the same value of physical properties as the irregularly shaped particle being studied. This particle diameter is in the literature also called equivalent diameter. Reference to the aerodynamic equivalent diameter of a particle is useful for describing settling and inertial behavior. Large particles, e.g., skin flakes, might have an inertial behavior similar to that of a particle with smaller aerodynamic diameter. The motion of a particle is of concern for impaction sampling devices (e.g., slit-to-agar samplers, sieve samplers, cascade samplers, and centrifugal samplers) and for settling plates.

SAMPLING EFFICIENCY

Physical Efficiency

The physical sampling efficiency of an aerosol sampler is influenced by inlet or extraction efficiency and by separation efficiency:

- Inlet or extraction efficiency is a function of the inlet design of the sampler and its ability to collect particles from the air in a representative way and transport the particles to the impaction nozzle or the filter.
- Separation efficiency is the ability of the sampling device to separate and collect particles of different sizes from the air stream by impaction onto the collection medium or into the filter medium.

The physical sampling efficiency is the same whether the particles consist of single microorganisms, carry microorganisms, or are nonviable (inanimate). The physical sampling efficiency is based on the physical characteristics of the sampling device such as airflow, orifice shape, and orifice size. The d_{50} (cutoff size) describes the aerodynamic equivalent particle diameter removed by 50% from the air stream and impacted. The d_{50}-value can, according to Hinds (2) and Nevalainen et al. (3), be calculated as follows:

$$d_{50} = \sqrt{\frac{9\eta D_h Stk_{50}}{\rho UC}} \tag{1}$$

where η is the viscosity of air [g/(cm·s)], D_h the hydraulic diameter of the air inlet nozzle (cm), Stk_{50} the Stokes number that gives 50% collection efficiency (nondimensional), ρ the particle density (g/cm³), U the impact velocity (cm/s), and C the Cunningham correction factor used for particles smaller than 1 µm (nondimensional).

Impactor collection data are usually given in terms of an aerodynamic d_{50} ($\rho = 1$ g/cm³) and the results of impactor measurements expressed in terms of aerodynamic diameter. The Cunningham correction factor could, for particle sizes discussed here, mostly be chosen as 1. For smaller particles and more accurate estimations, see Ref. (2). It could be mentioned that such a correction for particles with diameters of 1 and 0.5 µm, a reduction will occur with 8% and 14%, respectively. The Stk_{50} number is often chosen to 0.24 to 0.25 for inlet nozzles (2,3).

Most impaction sampling devices have sharp cutoff characteristics, meaning that almost all particles larger than that of d_{50} are collected.

However, it is not yet common for manufacturers of microbiological samplers to present the d_{50} of their equipment. Eq. (1) can be simplified using constant factors for air viscosity, particle density, and correction factor. The expression for d_{50} (in µm) will approximately become:

$$d_{50} \approx \sqrt{\frac{40D_h}{U}} \tag{2}$$

where D_h is the hydraulic diameter of the air inlet nozzle (mm) and U the impact velocity (m/s).

For a round opening, the hydraulic diameter D_h is the hole diameter. For a rectangular long slit (length much larger than the width), the hydraulic diameter will approximately be twice the slit width.

Examples

1. Calculate d_{50} for an impaction sampler with a sampling air volume flow of 100 L/min and a lid with 200 holes of diameter of 1 mm. The ratio between the airflow and the total hole area gives the impaction velocity of 10.6 m/s. With aid of eq. (2), the value of d_{50} will be estimated as 1.94 µm.
2. An impaction sampler with a sampling air volume flow of 50 L/min and a rectangular inlet slit 1 mm wide and 25 mm long has an impaction velocity of 33.3 m/s. The calculated d_{50} will, with the aid of eq. (2), be 1.55 µm.

Information of the d_{50}-value is an important factor when selecting the appropriate equipment for a cleanroom. However, the user should be aware that in a controlled environment with cleanroom dressed operators as main contamination source, the aerodynamic equivalent size of viable particles usually are smaller than in a typical operating theater. A study by Ljungqvist and Reinmüller (4) of the generation of viable particles from cleanroom dressed operators reported the viable particle size distribution according to results from the Andersen[R] 6-stage sampler (cascade sampler). The results shown as percentage of airborne aerobic colony forming units (CFUs) separated by the Andersen 6-stage sampler are illustrated in Figure 1.

Figure 1 shows that approximately one-third of the viable aerobic particles recovered are smaller than 2.1 µm according to the size distribution from Andersen 6-stage air sampler.

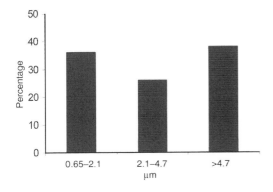

FIGURE 1 Viable aerodynamic particle size distribution in percent of airborne aerobic CFUs, measured with an Andersen 6-stage sampler (cascade sampler), during evaluation studies of operators dressed in new modern cleanroom clothing systems. *Abbreviation*: CFU, colony forming units. *Source*: From Ref. 4.

Biological Efficiency

The biological sampling efficiency, mostly below the physical sampling efficiency, is the ability to maintain the viability of the microorganisms during separation and collection in combination with the ability of the collection medium to support growth.

Guidance on the evaluation of biological efficiency is presented in the ISO 14698–1 (5) in the informative Annex B. The method described is based on a method by Clark et al. (6) and cannot be carried out in a common microbiological laboratory. The test should preferably be performed in an independent test laboratory. The results of the tests are expected to be provided by the manufacturer of the air sampler.

The method makes use of airborne particles of different sizes containing spores of *Bacillus subtilis* var. *niger* NCTC 10073 which survives the sampling conditions. To obtain the concentration of spores in the test chamber, a membrane filter is used. The concentration obtained from the test sampler is compared with the concentration from the membrane filter over five sizes between 0.8 and 15 µm. For each test, at least 10 experiments should be carried out. The efficiency of the tested sampler is calculated using the following equation:

$$\text{Efficiency of sampler}(\%) = \frac{\text{test sampler count}}{\text{total count (from membrane sampler)}} \times 100$$

(3)

Measuring the biological efficiency with microorganism typically found in the cleanroom is suggested as a better method by Whyte (7). Whyte also points out the importance of testing the air sampler including the tube extension if tube extensions are used.

AIR SAMPLING

General

Evaluation of environmental bioburden through the collection, recovery, and growth of airborne microorganisms is carried out using suitable sampling devices on a routine basis according to a defined sampling plan. One of the most common methods for clean zone bioburden evaluation is active air sampling.

There are three main methods for collecting particles that are used for micro-biological tests: impaction, filtration, and sedimentation. Impaction and filtration methods are considered active sampling techniques and require the collection of a known air volume. Sedimentation is the passive collection of airborne viable contamination by "fall out" or settling into an open Petri dish.

The purpose of the active sampling procedure is to separate particles from the air at a representative location without affecting the viability of the micro-organisms, and without altering the airflow pattern in the sampling region.

The selection of the most appropriate sampling device for a particular application depends upon the following factors:

■ Physical characteristics of the sampling equipment,
■ The type of viable particles to be sampled (single spores or cells that are carried by nonviable particles),
■ The equivalent size of particles to be collected,
■ The sensitivity of the viable particles to the sampling procedure,
■ The expected concentration of CFUs in the environment,
■ The ability to detect low levels of CFUs in a reliable way,
■ The time and duration of the sampling, and
■ The sampling location.

Furthermore, sampling in an aseptic environment requires that it is possible to sterilize or disinfect the sampling device and that the media, including the containers (plates or strips), are sterile. Aseptic skill in handling of the equipment is required. During operation of the sampler, particles equal to and larger than 0.5 μm should not be generated. Aerodynamic design of the device might be needed when sampling is performed within the critical zone. The relevance of a sampling location can be evaluated with the method for limitation of risks (LR method) described by Ljungqvist and Reinmüller (8). When using devices that create air wakes or turbulence, care must be taken especially, but not only, within the critical zone (9,10).

Active Sampling

There are several methods and devices available for the active collection of airborne viable particles. The purpose of the sampling should guide the selection of a particular method, material, and device. Airborne viable particulate sampling devices have been compared in several published studies (11–17).

ISO 14698–1 (5) considers air samplers that collect viable particulates by direct impact of particles on nutrient media and filtration samplers that collect particles on special filters suitable for active sampling in clean zones with a low biocontamination. The impaction velocity should be high enough to separate particles down to approximately 1 μm and low enough to avoid mechanical damage of the cells. For cleanrooms applications, 1 m³ should be sampled in a reasonable time without drying the collection medium.

Impaction

Impaction is the most commonly used technique for active air sampling. Impaction samplers increase the velocity of airborne particles by means of a hole, slit, or by a fan blade in the sampling head during the sampling. The stream of air is blown or drawn toward the surface of the collecting medium at high velocity. Because of inertia, the particles cannot follow the deflected air at the surface without being thrown against the surface and being caught on it (7,18). The cutoff size value d_{50} describes the aerodynamic size of impacting particles provided that the distance between the nozzle outlet and the collecting surface is suitably short. This distance should be greater than the hydraulic diameter of the nozzle opening. The upper value of this distance is not well known but it must be ensured that the air jet has not dissipated before impinging upon the plate. To produce a desirable sharp cutoff, the Reynolds number in the nozzle throat should be between 500 and 3000 (2,18). The collecting surface may consist of different sticky, solid materials such as agar media. The impaction principle is applied in different ways in slit-to-agar samplers, sieve samplers, and centrifugal samplers, each sampler with its own physical characteristics.

Filtration
Filtration constitutes a separation of particles on a filter. Membrane or depth-type filters can be used for microbiological air sampling. Particles penetrate into the filter and are retained and bound therein. The filter-bed material may be of a water-soluble substance that can be dissolved before culturing. With filtration methods, the risk of desiccation of the bacterial cells retained by the filter is of special concern. According to Jensen et al. (19), filtration is probably not a suitable method for evaluating the levels of vegetative cells due to its desiccating effects.

Passive Sampling
Particle sedimentation is the oldest collection technique. Passive microbial air sampling with settling plates (gravitational sedimentation sampling) is often used and is considered to give an estimate of the risk of contamination (20). The Annex 1 to the Guide to Good Manufacturing Practice for Medicinal Products (21) requires long-time monitoring of air in the grade A area [equivalent to the Food and Drug Administration (FDA) "critical area"] with settling plates in addition to the active sampling.

Settle Plates
The use of settling plates offers, because they are easy to handle and allow exposure times up to four hours, offers advantages over the more cumbersome active air sampling devices. The settling of particles onto the exposed plate is affected by local air movements, exposure time, and the particle settling velocity.

POINTS TO CONSIDER
It is generally accepted that the estimation of the concentration of airborne CFUs can be affected by the choice of sampler, agar volume of collection containers, and the sampling method. Available sampling devices have characteristics that make them more or less suitable for use in a specific environment, or for a specific type of sampling.

Different strategies for environmental monitoring might be applied for different processing conditions. Qualification of cleanrooms, routine monitoring, or trouble shooting each requires a specific approach. The use of risk analysis systems during assessment of microbiological hazards in cleanrooms is a recommendation (5).

The monitoring program should have a scientifically based sampling plan, which considers sampling methods and devices, locations, and frequencies. The rationale for each sampling location should be clear. In addition, control levels should be established along with the actions to be taken when results exceed these preset levels. If a great number of manual interventions are required during manufacturing operations, the importance of the environmental monitoring program increases.

The locations for air sampling should be determined during the commissioning/qualification and start-up of a cleanroom or controlled environment. Considerations should be given to the proximity to the product and whether air might be in contact with a product. It may be prudent to identify indicator sites, which are near but not in contact with the product. Locations with intensive personnel movement or high population of staff should be considered as critical areas for monitoring.

An environmental control program should refer to validated methods, and the devices used for active air sampling should be characterized and calibrated.

Once the appropriate media and sampling volume have been selected with regard to regulatory requirements, specific contamination risks to the process, and the design of the sampler, the incubation time and temperature can be chosen. Incubation time and temperature may vary depending upon the predominant types of microflora or upon the selected media. The incubation time should be long enough to ensure the growth of recovered microorganisms. By experience, three days at 30°C to 35°C are a minimum for mesophilic bacteria. Fungi might require two to four additional days of incubation at room temperature in daylight. The sterility of the media and its container is critical. Media sterilization processes must be validated and the media must be tested for sterility and for growth promotion prior to or concurrent with its use.

Microbial monitoring need not always identify all microbial contaminants present in controlled environments. However, routine monitoring should provide enough information so that adequate remedial actions can be taken if contamination levels exceed control levels. In order that decisions can be made regarding corrective actions, identification of isolates to the genus or in some cases species level is required for tracing a contamination. The methods used for identification of isolates should be validated with known microorganisms as well as with the most common isolates from the environment being monitored. Control organisms used to validate microbial identification methods should be traceable to recognized type culture collections, such as American Type Culture Collection. Subcultures taken from type culture stocks should not be more than five serial passages from the master stock to ensure purity and identity.

SUMMARY

To interpret the results from viable air sampling, the user should understand the dynamics of sampling and collection of viable particles on the collection medium. Results of 0 CFU/m^3 in manned cleanrooms could indicate that the sampling process, sampling location or the collection media, incubation time, and temperature have not been optimized.

It is important to be aware of the limitations of each sampling method. Results achieved with one method must not be compared with results from another method without careful investigation. To improve the evaluation of controlled environments based on achieved results, the air sampler used has to be specified. An air sampler must be selected based on a careful evaluation of the sampler's characteristics, the sampling conditions, and sampling requirements.

Systematic, purposeful, and economic microbiological monitoring of airborne contaminants is the goal. The rational of each sampling location should be clear. When necessary, a sampling location should be evaluated with regard to its response to detect nonaccepted interventions in critical zones.

Trending should be performed with regard to the concentration of CFUs, frequency of detected growth, and to the identified species within the total environmental monitoring for the respective area. Microbiological results from air, surfaces, people, and results from continuous particle monitoring should be evaluated together.

The microbiological contamination in air varies highly with the activity in the sampling region and the sampling time usually is relatively short; the active sampling techniques give only limited information about the concentration of viable particles in the cleanroom at a specified time and no indications of conditions before or after sampling.

Particle monitoring cannot be considered a substitute for microbial monitoring, as it does not provide adequate information regarding the presence of viable particles. However, continuous monitoring of airborne particles provides information regarding total airborne particle levels during specific work activities, and the length of clean up periods within the clean environment. When this information is combined with the results from the routine monitoring of airborne viable particles in the cleanroom, a relationship might be established between the number of total airborne particles equal to and larger than $0.5\,\mu m$ per volume unit of air and the number of airborne CFUs per volume unit of air. This relation is probably similar for cleanrooms with a high degree of uniformity regarding processes and number of people present.

A real-time measurement technique using particle counters provides the ability to immediately detect changes in the cleanroom. Current good manufacturing practice (GMP) asks for periodic or continuous monitoring at representative locations to be carried out during dynamic manufacturing conditions. The results should be evaluated promptly to detect deviations from normally observed levels. Increased concentrations indicate increased activity in the cleanroom and should be noted by the microbiologist evaluating the air samples from the same time. Particle monitoring is a valuable tool for the systematic evaluation of changes, whether those changes reduce or increase process risks.

To base the risk assessment on environmental monitoring data requires an understanding of the process, the cleanroom, and environmental microbiology. To know what and when deviations imply hazardous conditions and a risk to the products requires both technological and microbiological experiences.

REFERENCES

1. Willeke K, Baron PA, eds. Aerosol Measurement: Principles, Techniques and Applications. New York: Van Nostrand Reinhold, 1993.
2. Hinds WC. Aerosol Technology. 2nd ed. New York: Wiley, 1999.
3. Nevalainen A, Willeke K, Liebhaber F, Pastuszka J, Burge H, Henningson E. Bioaerosol sampling. In: Willeke K, Baron PA, eds. Aerosol Measurement: Principles, Techniques and Applications. New York: Van Nostrand Reinhold, 1993:471–492.
4. Ljungqvist B, Reinmüller B. Cleanroom Clothing Systems, People as a Contamination Source. Bethesda, MD; PDA/River Grove, IL: DHI Publishing LLC, 2004.
5. ISO 14698-1. Cleanrooms and associated controlled environments—Biocontamination control—Part 1: General Principles and Methods. Geneva: International Organization for Standards, 2003.
6. Clark S, Lach V, Lidwell OM. The performance of the Biotest RCS centrifugal air sampler. J Hosp Infect 1981; 2:181–186.
7. Whyte W. Collection efficiency of microbial methods used to monitor cleanrooms. Eur J Parenter Pharmaceut Sci 2005; 10(2):43–50.
8. Ljungqvist B, Reinmüller B. Hazard analyses of airborne contamination in cleanrooms—application of a method for limitation of risks. PDA J Pharmaceut Sci Technol 1995; 49:239–243.
9. Ljungqvist B, Reinmüller B. Some aspects on the use of the biotest RCS air sampler in unidirectional air flow testing. J Parenter Sci Technol 1991; 45(4):177–180.
10. Ljungqvist B, Reinmüller B. The Biotest RCS air sampler in unidirectional flow. J Pharm Sci Technol 1994; 48(1):41–44.
11. Vogt KH. Quantitative Keimzahlbestimmung in der Raumluft—Zwei Geräte und Methoden im Vergleich. In: Krankenhaus-Hygiene + Infektionsverhütung. Heidelberg: Verlag für Medicin Dr. Ewald Fischer GmbH, 1990; 12:34–37.
12. Hecker W, Meier R. Bestimmung der Luftkeimzahl im Produktionsbereich mit neurem Geräten. Pharm Ind 1991; 53(5):496–503.
13. Benbough JE, Bennett AM, Parks SR. Determination of the collection efficiency of a microbial air sampler. J Appl Bacteriol 1993; 74:170–173.
14. Willeke K, Grinshpun SA, Donnelly J, et al. Physical and biological sampling efficiencies of bioaerosol samplers. In: Indoor Air '93. Proceedings of the Sixth International Conference on Indoor Air Quality and Climate, Helsinki, Vol. 4, 1993:131–136.
15. Griffiths WD, DeCosemo GAL. The assessment of bioaerosols: a critical review. J Aerosol Sci 1994; 25(8):1425–1458.
16. Henningson EW, Ahlberg MS. Evaluation of microbiological aerosol samplers: a review. J Aerosol Sci 1994; 25:1459–1492.
17. Ljungqvist B, Reinmüller B. Active sampling of airborne viable particles in controlled environments: a comparative study of common instruments. Eur J Parenter Sci 1998; 3(3):59–62.
18. Marple VA, Rubow KL, Olson BA. Inertial, gravitational, centrifugal and thermal collection techniques. In: Willeke K, Baron PA, eds. Aerosol Measurement: Principles, Techniques and Applications. New York: Van Nostrand Reinhold, 1993:206–232.
19. Jensen PA, Todd WF, Davis GN, Scarpino PV. Evaluation of eight bioaerosol samplers challenged with aerosols of free bacteria. Am Ind Hyg Assoc J 1992; 53(10):660–667.
20. Whyte W. Sterility assurance and models for assessing airborne bacterial contamination. J Parenter Sci Technol 1986; 40(5):188–197.
21. EU GMP European Commission. The Rules Governing Medicinal Products in the European Community. Vol. IV. Guide to Good Manufacturing Practice, incl. Annex 1, Manufacture of Sterile Medicinal Products. 1997 revised 2003.

5 Microbial Surface Monitoring

Scott Sutton

5 Microbial Surface Monitoring

Scott Sutton

Vectech Pharmaceutical Consultants, Farmington Hills, Michigan, U.S.A.

INTRODUCTION

The accurate and consistent microbial monitoring of controlled rooms as a measure of quality control is an important measure in the manufacture of sterile and non-sterile pharmaceutical products. While it is a direct measure of the bioburden in the environment immediately surrounding the product manufacture, it cannot be overinterpreted as a measure of finished product quality (1), but rather a measure of the state of control of the facility and operations. Other chapters in this book deal with the importance of air-monitoring techniques; it is the purpose of this chapter to present the methods for microbial monitoring of surfaces. From the outset, we have to note that the link between surface sampling results, viable air monitoring, and personnel monitoring is a basic assumption of the industry, one that has never been demonstrated (2,3). In fact, recent data designed to test this assumption call its validity into question (4).

In addition to the methods themselves, we will discuss the means to determine the sampling efficiency of the methods. Determination of the sampling efficiency of the method is a required parameter of method validation. Another critical parameter for both the validation and the performance of the test is the determination of the uncertainty of the method used. Finally, we will briefly examine some potential alternatives to traditional microbiological methods in this area, as there are large advantages to the manufacture available from reducing the timelines for product manufacture and release.

Regulatory Requirements

Although directed specifically at aseptic processing, the Food and Drug Administration (FDA) guide to aseptic processing (5) describes the importance for environmental monitoring for all manufacturing conditions:

> In aseptic processing, one of the most important laboratory controls is the environmental-monitoring program. This program provides meaningful information on the quality of the aseptic processing environment (e.g., when a given batch is being manufactured) as well as environmental trends of ancillary clean areas. Environmental monitoring should promptly identify potential routes of contamination, allowing for implementation of corrections before product contamination occurs (211.42 and 211.113).
>
> Evaluating the quality of air and surfaces in the cleanroom environment should start with a well-defined written program and scientifically sound methods. The monitoring program should cover all production shifts and include air, floors, walls, and equipment surfaces, including the critical surfaces that come in contact with the product, container, and closures. Written procedures should include a list of locations to be sampled. Sample timing, frequency, and location should be carefully selected based upon their relationship to the operation

performed. Samples should be taken throughout the classified areas of the aseptic processing facility (e.g., aseptic corridors, gowning rooms) using scientifically sound sampling procedures. Sample sizes should be sufficient to optimize detection of environmental contaminants at levels that might be expected in a given clean area.

There are then two overriding concerns in monitoring; that the monitoring provide meaningful information on product quality, and that the sampling methods be scientifically sound. We will examine the subject of surface-monitoring procedures from these two perspectives in this chapter.

Overall, there can be little controversy over the advisability of conducting microbial assays as part of the control tests on the manufacturing process (6). A major concern in sterile product manufacture is the absence of microorganisms. However, there is legitimate concern that the current regulatory climate encourages the distressing trend to overinterpret the microbiology data and apply the testing methods inappropriately (5,7).

Personnel

Monitoring of personnel in the aseptic environment is an important factor in both demonstrating adequate control and maintaining documentation of that compliance on the part of the operators. The largest source of contamination in a cleanroom is the personnel working there (8), therefore containment of that contamination by the aseptic gowns is of paramount importance to prevent shedding of particulate contamination into the air and to prevent contamination of material through touch. Personnel monitoring provides documentation as to the state of control of the operators.

A second major advantage of this monitoring is that it is also an excellent mechanism to constantly remind the operators of the importance of microbial concerns. Many companies place pass/fail criteria on personnel monitoring results, and an employee's access to the aseptic core can be revoked for exceeding the acceptance criteria for this monitoring.

Barrier Isolators

While there is room for a reasonable debate on the utility of environmental monitoring inside a barrier isolator unit, there is clear regulatory expectation that this monitoring will occur. Appendix 1 of the FDA aseptic processing guide (4) explicitly states "an appropriate environmental-monitoring program should be established that routinely ensures acceptable microbiological quality of air, surfaces, and gloves (or half-suits) as well as particle levels, within the isolator."

The Pharmaceutical Inspection Convention and Pharmaceutical Inspection Co-operation Scheme (PIC/S) Guidance document on isolators (9) provides some excellent cautionary notes on this topic:

> 9.5.7.2 Microbiological monitoring should take into account the special requirements for sensitivity of testing in isolators subjected to a sporicidal process and avoid compromising operations. The interpretation of results of environmental monitoring should be based on the premise that the detection of any microbiological contamination probably indicates a failure of the system.
> 9.5.7.2.1 Media fills and sterility testing should be carried out as normal for aseptic processing.
> 9.5.7.2.2 Environmental monitoring within the isolator should not interfere with zone protection, and in process controls should not carry any risk for production.

9.5.7.2.3 The use of settle plates, contact plates, swabs and the presence of sampling points for active air samplers or particle counters may add risk to the system subjected to a sporicidal process. Some of the ways that this may be addressed include the following:

- Sampling at the end of production.
- Sampling at potentially worst case positions, e.g., in an exhaust.
- Using multiple wrapped irradiated plates and swabs etc. may reduce the risk of introducing contamination into the system, but there have been instances when the supplier has made changes or mistakes and compromised processes. The fertility of irradiated media should be given special attention. Testing the supplier's formula at extremes of the irradiation treatment using local isolates as well as standard cultures should be considered. The effect of exposure of wrapped plates, etc. to the sporicidal process should be examined in case of loss of fertility due to penetration of the agent.
- A significant risk to the interpretation of results is the accidental infection of plates etc. by subsequent handling, so incubation in sealed sterile pass out bags may be necessary. Another risk to the interpretation of results is the presence of a colony that developed prior to irradiation.
- Built in sampling systems should be gassed or otherwise assured to be free from contamination and not compromise operations, special arrangements of filters and/or valves may be used.
- Quantitative results are not as relevant as in conventional clean rooms because the detection of any contamination probably indicates something has failed. Conventional sampling may be replaced by 'in house' devices known to be sterile, such as settling pots full of media or transport fluid. Large areas of the gloves and isolator surfaces may be swabbed and the swab incubated in sterile broth.

Demonstration Cleaning/Disinfection Efficacy

Surface monitoring is vital as a component in the demonstration of adequate cleaning/disinfection program (10–12). The best evidence a facility can have of the appropriate selection of disinfectants, procedures, and application is the continued documentation of surface monitoring results that are under control. Although the concern of microorganisms developing resistance to biocides and overrunning the facility is not scientifically supportable (13), different species of bacteria can and do display different sensitivities to biocidal agents. A major problem in this regard is the presence of spore-forming microorganisms that can survive biocide application designed to destroy vegetative microorganisms. Exclusive use of a disinfectant may result in the accumulation of spore-forming microorganisms. Continued monitoring of the facility surfaces, with identification of the organisms seen, can be extremely useful in determining when a sporicidal agent should be used in addition to (or in place of) the standard cleaning regimen (14).

Sample Sites

The sample sites must be chosen with care in any aspect of the environmental-monitoring program, surface sites are no exception. Prior to choosing the sites to include in a validation protocol, a thorough study of the facility, the work flow, and the product contact and product exposure areas should be made. The sites for the validation study are chosen to "overtest" the area. Once the data have been collected for a number of weeks, the sites can be evaluated for their proximity to

TABLE 1 Levels Provided in Common References—Surface Viables (Except Floors)

Regional standard	Class (limit)	Class (limit)	Class (limit)
USP <1116>	M3.5 (3 CFU/contact plate)	M5.5 (5 CFU/contact plate)	M6.5 (not stated)
EU; at rest, static	A and B (not stated)	C (not stated)	D (not stated)
EU; operational, dynamic	A (<1 CFU/contact plate)	C (25 CFU/contact plate)	D (50 CFU/contact plate)
EU; operational, dynamic	B (5 CFU/contact plate)	C (25 CFU/contact plate)	D (50 CFU/contact plate)

Abbreviations: CFU, colony-forming units; USP, United States Pharmacopeia; EU, European Union.

open product (and so potential for product contamination) and for the frequency and degree of contamination seen. This consideration is important to provide as sensitive a measure as possible for the state of facility control (15).

Trending and Control

One of the major advantages to collecting data over a period of time is the ability to trend and analyze the data from a historical perspective. This trending is certainly expected from regulatory agencies (4) and is recommended by United States Pharmacopeia (USP) (16). While the traditional method of setting alert and action levels is to determine specific plate counts of interest, this method is not supportable given the limitations of the measurement method.

The traditional method of setting alert and action levels is by the observance of specific levels. Levels that are in the literature are presented in Table 1(surface), Table 2 (gowns), and Table 3 (gloves) (17). While these levels are recognized by regulatory agencies, they may not be appropriate for a specific location and situation. It is strongly recommended to conduct periodic reviews of the historical data for all environmental-monitoring data and evaluate the trends, not limiting your evaluation to the arbitrary levels found in regulatory guidance (4).

Another philosophy on setting levels is that you should use the historical data to determine reasonable levels for your facility. This is complicated by the fact that most control charts are based on data following a normal distribution, while microbiological data follow a Poisson distribution (18,19). However, these data can be evaluated using different methods (20,21).

An alternate trending method that is gaining acceptance is to determine a frequency model that provides useful indication of the facility's state of control. In

TABLE 2 Levels Provided in Common References—Personnel Gowns

Regional standard	Class (limit)	Class (limit)	Class (limit)
USP <1116>	M3.5 (5 CFU/contact plate)	M5.5 (20 CFU/contact plate)	M6.5 (not stated)
EU; at rest, static	A and B (not stated)	C (not stated)	D (not stated)
EU; operational, dynamic	A (<1 CFU/contact plate)	C (25 CFU/contact plate)	D (50 CFU/contact plate)
EU; operational, dynamic	B (5 CFU/contact plate)	C (25 CFU/contact plate)	D (50 CFU/contact plate)

Abbreviations: CFU, colony-forming units; USP, United States Pharmacopeia; EU, European Union.

TABLE 3 Levels Provided in Common References—Personnel Gloves

Regional standard	Class (limit)	Class (limit)	Class (limit)
USP <1116>	M3.5 (3 CFU/contact plate)	M5.5 (10 CFU/contact plate)	M6.5 (not stated)
EU; at rest, static	A and B (not stated)	C (not stated)	D (not stated)
EU; operational, dynamic	A (<1 CFU/glove, print of five fingers)	C (not stated)	D (not stated)
EU; operational, dynamic	B (<1 CFU/glove, print of five fingers)	C (not stated)	D (not stated)

Abbreviation: CFU, colony-forming unit.

this method, the absolute number of organisms collected from a particular site is less important than the frequency of isolation. This method is particularly attractive in testing the highly controlled areas of an aseptic facility, where the expectation is to recover no colony-forming units (CFU) per plate. On occurrences where some recovery occurs, distinguishing between 1 CFU (pass) and 3 CFU (fail) may not be a scientifically supportable distinction (7).

Assistance in Investigation

A final aspect of the environmental-monitoring program and surface monitoring that must be addressed is the assistance it may offer in a product test investigation (FDA 2004). Note that we are not discussing the controversial practice of treating environmental-monitoring excursions as "out-of-specification" (OOS) events requiring a full investigation, although that approach also has support (22). The practice of conducting OOS investigations on surface monitoring and environmental excursions implies that these excursions are as indicative of compromised product quality as is a product release test, which is clearly not the case (23).

However, trending information, and the identification of microorganisms associated with surface monitoring, can be extremely useful in an investigation of a finished product release test failure. It can be particularly useful if a particular organism can be traced through the product process as the causative agent of the compromised product quality.

TYPES OF MONITORING METHODS

The method of testing will have a direct impact on the number of organisms seen. The choice of monitoring method at a specific site, therefore, can have a direct impact on the environmental-monitoring validation plan and the ability of the facility to demonstrate a state of control. In choosing the method, it is important to consider the type of material to be tested and the classification of the cleanroom itself.

It will be useful to examine the different methods to monitor surfaces before describing the validation concerns, as well as discussing the different methods of determining the efficiencies of the sampling methods. Many types of methods have been developed (24), but most are not in common usage in the pharmaceutical industry. The two most commonly used are the contact plate [or replicate organism detection and counting (RODAC)] and swabbing (25,26), used by virtually all manufacturers. The RODAC contact plate method is more suitable to flat, firm surfaces while the swab is more useful for flexible, uneven, or heavily contaminated surfaces (27).

RODAC Plates

The RODAC plate was first described by Hall and Hartnett (28) as a means of direct sampling for surface contamination. It has become widely accepted due to its ease of use and wide applicability. The method employs small Petri dishes (surface area of approximately 25 cm^2), overfilled with nutrient agar. The surface tension of the molten nutrient agar holds the liquid in place, projecting beyond the upper edge of the dish as the agar sets (29). The contact plate is then used by pressing it against the flat surface to be tested. Organisms on the surface of the equipment will be lifted off and remain adherent to the agar. The RODAC plate is then covered and incubated, with the CFU/plate reported (30).

This method is used not only for sampling of flat surfaces of equipment but also for personnel. A variant on this method is the touch plate where personnel will place their fingertips on the surface of an agar plate to get an estimate of the number of microorganisms on the tips.

There are several limitations to this method (31). The most obvious is the need for a flat surface as the agar projecting above the dish must come into contact with the surface being tested. A second limitation is that this method is very sensitive to residual disinfectant that may be on the surface and transferred, although this limitation can be overcome by incorporation of neutralizing agents into the nutrient agar (32,33).

Other limitations of the method are common for any of the enumeration methods. To derive numbers, we are forced to use the measurement of CFU as determined by growth in or on agar. The number of CFUs has a lower limit of quantification, normally recognized to be at 25 CFU/plate (34). At the other extreme, the linear range of CFU/plate is considered to be around 250 CFU for a standard sized plate (35). The smaller size of the Petri dish implies a smaller range (i.e., a lower upper limit to the countable number of colonies on the plate). Finally, as this method involves direct contact between the nutrient agar and the surface being tested, media residue remaining on the surface must be removed.

Swab

Swabs can be used in those situations where the use of contact plate is impractical, i.e., to test irregular surfaces. A moistened swab (typically cotton, Dacron, or calcium alginate) is used to scrub the surface after which the microorganisms are resuspended in a buffer and plated (or filtered, then plated) for recovery and determination of CFU (36). This method is somewhat operator dependent (37), but can serve well in those situations where the RODAC plate cannot be used.

The swab material type can have an effect on the recovery. Rose et al. (38) evaluated four swab materials for the recovery of *Bacillus anthracis* spores from steel coupons and found that premoistened (rather than dry) macrofoam and cotton swabs had far better recovery of the artificially inoculated steel coupons than did polyester or rayon swabs. Care must always be taken in interpreting these studies, of course, as the recovery efficiencies are heavily influenced by the method used and data from challenge studies may not reflect data generated from naturally contaminated surfaces. Another common material type, calcium alginate, also can be useful as the entire sampling material can be brought into solution so that the microorganisms could be recovered by filtration.

The swab method has a large number of manipulations in comparison to the RODAC method. After sampling and transport to the lab, microorganisms from the swab are resuspended, filtered, the filter is placed on a nutrient agar surface, and then the sample in incubated for growth. This process calls for strict adherence to aseptic technique by the operator to avoid accidental contamination.

Another consideration when evaluating recovery methods is the potential for the choice of method to influence the type of organisms recovered. For example, the swab technique might recover a different range of bacteria than the RODAC. Lemmen et al. (39) conducted an in-use evaluation of the two methods in the hospital environment. Over a period of 22 months, the two methods were used side-by-side in hospital rooms. They found gram-positive cocci more often than gram-negative bacteria overall, and found that RODAC plates gave higher recoveries of the gram-positive organisms. The swab technique was more effective at recovering gram-negative rods than was the RODAC method. All results were statistically significant.

Surface Rinse

In general terms, the surface rinse method involves vigorously agitating sterile liquid over the surface to be tested, then recovering the liquid, filtering the recovered liquid, laying the membrane filter on a nutrient agar plate, and then incubating for growth. One application for this technology is to sample the interior of large equipment.

It would be very difficult to get a technician to the interior of some sterile equipment to conduct surface sampling for microbial contamination. However, the technician could introduce sterile water into that space, agitate, and then recover the test solution for further evaluation. This method allows sampling in areas that would be impossible by other means. However, it also involves a large number of physical manipulations, any one of which could introduce contamination into the sample leading to erroneous results. Great care in aseptic technique is necessary to successfully employ this technique.

Other Sampling Methods

There are many other types of methods described in the literature from the food, clinical, and applied microbiology literature. Few have acceptance in the pharmaceutical industry due to concerns over contamination of cleanrooms and the need for strict aseptic handling. Several of these methods are described here.

Flexible Films

The concept behind the commercially available flexible film sampling devices is that they try to retain the positive attributes of the RODAC plate, while allowing some sampling of modestly irregular surfaces. The nutrient agar is placed on a flexible foil backing, allowing sampling of curved surfaces. After sampling, the agar is incubated and the colonies counted as for the contact plate.

Agar Sausage

The basic method involves creating nutrient agar cylinders—the original author made them in artificial sausage casings, hence the name (40). The end of the "sausage" is cut off to make a smooth surface, then the smooth end placed on the surface to be sampled. The sample is then cut off, placed in a sterile Petri dish, and the newly exposed end can be used for another sampling event. Periodically sausage ends can be cut off to check for sterility. The disadvantages associated with manipulations of this type are obvious.

Direct Agar Overlay

This method was developed to provide a means for comparison of commonly used recovery methods (41). In principle, a circle is drawn on a tile of the nonporous surface to be tested using a wax pencil (the authors used the bottom of a Petri dish to make a circle approximately 4.0 in.^{2}). Nutrient agar is poured into the circle and allowed to solidify. The agar is then covered with a Petri dish cover (containing a piece of moistened filter paper to retard drying) and incubated in a high-humidity incubator at 35°C overnight. The agar is then flooded with a dye (2,3,5-triphenyl 2H-tetrazolium chloride was used) until the colonies turned deep red. The tile was then dried for 10 to 15 minutes at 65°C to 70°C. The colonies were then counted under slight magnification. This method is obviously not suitable for use in a cleanroom, but might find application as a control study on method qualification investigations.

Membrane Filter Sampling

Nitrocellulose membrane filters have been suggested as a sampling device for surface sampling (42). This method has been evaluated in comparison with RODAC plate sampling and found to compare favorably (43). The basic technique is to take a sterile nitrocellulose membrane, place it in contact with the surface to be tested (for approximately 30 sec) and then place it on the surface of a nutrient agar plate or pad soaked in nutrient medium (sample side up). The colonies are directly read from the surface of the membrane following incubation.

The study of Poletti et al. (43) was extensively controlled for sampling variability by design and used a glass surface contaminated by 24 hour exposure to air in an animal facility. Multiple samples were taken from different locations on the glass by each method, and the resultant counts were compared statistically. In this study, the nitrocellulose filter sampling method was more effective than RODAC plates.

An earlier study on the use of membrane filters provided some interesting observations on nominal pore size effects (44). The authors were concerned with the sampling of burn sites for clinical evaluation, and so were looking to recovery from moist samples. They artificially inoculated two test materials: the bottom of Petri dishes and bovine skeletal muscle. The inoculum was laboratory-prepared bacterial suspensions, sampled within five minutes. Using this method, the membrane filter technique was effective, with the 5 μm membrane giving better results than the 0.45, 1.2, or 3 μm pore rated membranes. Unfortunately, the authors of this study did not indicate the membrane material type.

Foam Sampling Device

The BisKit is a single-use device that allows the sampling of a 1 m^2 area at a single time. The kit contains a resuspension buffer that is forced through the foam after sampling and is then collected for membrane filtration and determination of the colony numbers on the membrane surface. Due to the large sample size, a great deal greater sensitivity is possible. However, this large sample size also reduces the number of sites where the technique may be used and increases the residue issues. In addition, the kit, while commercially available, comes at a high cost per test. However, this kit has been shown to be very efficient at recovery of spores artificially seeded onto common building material (45).

Spray/Suspension

Clark (46) described a spray method for the rinsing of microbes off the surface of a wall. The method used a spray gun with a dedicated cup and collection device.

The sterile water, sprayed on the wall and collected, was then evaluated for viable cells by membrane filtration. The requirements for sterile change parts (sprayer, cup, collection device) has hindered acceptance of this method.

A similar concept is the collection cylinder. In this method, a hollow cylinder of known circumference is placed on a horizontal, smooth surface. Sampling buffer is added to the cylinder, filling it part way. The liquid is then agitated, and then removed to a sterile collection tube by pipette. The liquid is filtered and the membrane places on nutrient agar for microbial recovery. This method has been described for the evaluation of skin microbes (47).

These methods suffer from excessive manipulations, the requirement for a significant number of different sterile consumables, and significant residue on the sample surface after testing. In addition, they are limited to very small numbers of different surface types (the Clark apparatus to smooth walls, the cylinder to smooth horizontal surfaces).

Agar Slides

The agar slide is a variant of the contact plate that has been used in the food industry. One of the most popular commercial varieties is the Hygcult TPC dipslide. The slide comes prepackaged in a screw-cap tube, with the solid agar support attached to the cap at a hinge. The sample is taken by holding the cap and pressing the agar flat onto the surface to be tested.

Salo et al. (48) reported on a 12-laboratory collaborative study using stainless steel coupons and artificially inoculated laboratory strains. They allowed drying of the challenge suspensions for five minutes (at which time they report standing liquid on the coupon remained) and then tested the dipslide, RODAC plating, and swabbing. The dipslide performed as well as the contact plate and swabbing.

EFFICACY OF METHODS

The validation of sampling methods requires some estimation of the sampling efficiency of the method on the materials found in your facility. To qualify or validate the method, there must be some way to estimate the numbers of organisms removed as a percentage of the total microorganisms (49).

ISO EN 1175–1996 (50) provides three criteria for validation of microbial recovery:

1. Assessment of the adequacy of the technique used to remove micro-organisms from the product, if such removal is part of the technique; and
2. assessment of the adequacy of the technique used to enumerate removed microorganisms, including microbiological counting techniques and culture conditions; and
3. assessment of the recovery efficiency of the method used in order that the correction factor can be calculated.

Although the specific guidance document addresses bioburden of medical devices, the philosophy captured in first and second points is valid for all studies of this type. ISO 11737–1 extends this consideration to the production process (51). The validation also needs to take into account the particular strengths and weaknesses of the method being validated and determine the appropriateness of that measure. These concerns are equally applicable to surface-monitoring studies. A good review of the different methods and validation concerns is provided by Favero et al. (52).

The choice of method to conduct the microbial monitoring will affect the validation design, as will the choice of which method to use to analyze the data. However, before making these decisions it is important to at least briefly examine the nature of organisms on a surface.

Nature of Microorganisms on a Surface

Microbial surface contamination may come from several sources. In highly controlled areas, the main source of microbial load will be from the operators, and can be assumed to be associated with skin flakes. However, in sampling from the rest of the facility, there can be many different types of adherence mechanisms holding the endogenous bioburden to the cleanroom surfaces (53). These mechanisms can include electrostatic mechanisms, metabolic mechanisms mediated initially by the pili of the cell, then by production of an extracellular glycocalyx, or a variety of other means. The association of microorganisms with a solid matrix is rarely one of the bacteria laying there, a factor that complicates validation studies.

A second factor that complicates these studies is the difficulty of getting a reproducible inoculum on the surface. A common approach is to grow a challenge organism inoculum in the lab, then lay the bacterial suspension of the material to be tested. If the material is allowed to dry, the cells become desiccated and die (54,55), usually at unpredictable levels. One way around this issue is to test the surface before it is completely dry, but it is unclear if this method is addressing the ability of the method to sample from the surface or the ability of the method to sample cells in suspension. A second way around the problem of desiccation is to use microbial spores, which are naturally resistant to death by desiccation. This approach, however, is divorced from the actual conditions to be tested as it only measures the ability of the method to recover spores laid across the surface. A final method is to naturally contaminate the material, and then repeatedly sample the same location. Eventually no more bacteria will be recovered and it is assumed that after repeated sampling to extinction, all microorganisms on the surface were recovered. These examine the validation methods in detail.

Validation by Repetitive Recovery

ISO 111737–1 (51) describes a method of repetitive recovery to validate the sampling method. The principle of this method is that the method of sampling should be repeated on the same location until there is no more recovery. Recovery efficiency is determined in this method by dividing the initial recovery by the sum of all CFU recovered.

This assumes that the material has a bioburden, that cells are not dying off as the sampling is occurring, that no further contamination of the site is occurring, that you have sampled sufficiently to exhaust the bioburden, and that all bioburden is removed. It has the advantage of using native bioburden in a normal state of adherence rather than artificially inoculated organisms. Annex B of this ISO 111737–1 describes the method in detail.

Linear Regression Method

Whyte (56) presented a linear regression method that is very similar to the method outlined above. Rather than calculating the recovery efficiency using only the two data points (initial and total recovery), this method uses all the numbers generated. This method provides a much more accurate estimate, but suffers from the same requirements as the method described above for repetitive recovery, with the

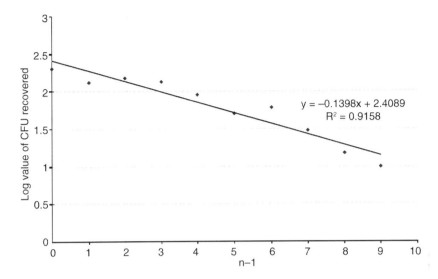

FIGURE 1 Example data for replicate organism detection and counting recovery efficiency. *Abbreviation*: CFU, colony-forming unit.

additional assumption that all microorganisms on the surface adhere with the same tenacity through the sampling events (the use of linear regression assumes linearity).

First of all, the CFU/sampling event is converted to the $\log_{10}$ value (the data transformation converts the numbers to approximate a normal distribution) (Table 4). Then linear regression analysis is performed of the sample number (independent variable) and the $\log_{10}$ CFU obtained (dependent variable). The sampling efficiency is determined from the liner regression equation of $Y = mX + C$, where m is the slope of the line and is equal to $\log_{10}(1 - \text{sampling efficiency})$.

An example is given here: Data from a RODAC sampling experiment (Fig. 1) Linear regression:[a]

$$y = -0.1398x + 2.4089 \text{ with a correlation coefficient } R_2 = 0.9158$$

Analysis:

Slope $= m = -0.1398 = \log_{10}(1 - \text{sampling efficiency})$.
Sampling efficiency $= 1 - 10^m = 1 - 0.27523 = 0.27523 = 27\%$.

In comparison, the previous method gives a recovery efficiency of

$$\text{Recovery} - \frac{200}{868} - 0.230415 - 23\%.$$

This method was also used by Yamayoshi et al. (57) to demonstrate the use of swabbing as a microbial recovery method in areas of very high contamination. The authors argued that in their hands, the measured rate of removal was almost constant among all the materials tested, and so proposed a single number for all swabbing efficiency calculations. It should be noted that this single efficiency number has not been verified by others and that it is recommended that all monitoring studies be validated.

---

[a] Note that the dependent variable in this analysis is $(n-1)$, not n itself.

TABLE 4

Sample number (n)	$n-1$	Count	$\log_{10}$ count
1	0	200	2.30103
2	1	130	2.113943
3	2	150	2.176091
4	3	134	2.127105
5	4	89	1.94939
6	5	50	1.69897
7	6	60	1.778151
8	7	30	1.477121
9	8	15	1.176091
10	9	10	1

Another treatment of this method can be found in the article by Eginton (58) who used this linear regression method to analyze removal of microorganisms from artificially inoculated tiles. They found significant differences in efficiencies depending on organism tested and tile material.

Through this method, typical recovery efficiencies for contact plates and swabs are commonly found in the range of 15% to 35% when using naturally contaminated material. The major disadvantage to this method is the challenge inherent in creating contaminated surfaces to test. The method of contamination that will yield representative bioburden on the surface is difficult to standardize.

Validation Using Inoculated Product

Annex B of ISO 11737–1 discusses a second method to validate microbial recovery. In this method, a challenge organism is used to inoculate the surface with a known number of microorganisms (spores of *Bacillus subtilis* var. *niger* are recommended for convenience and resistance to desiccation). The number of organisms removed with one sample is divided by the number inoculated (taking into consideration the surface area sampled) to provide the recovery efficiency.

The use of inoculated material is also recommended by the Parenteral Drug Association. Technical Report #21 entitled "Bioburden Recovery Validation" examines both medical device and surface-monitoring methods (59). The use of several artificial inocula is recommended, including bacterial vegetative cells and spores, yeast, and mold. Although mention is made in the technical report of the problem of inocula desiccation, no acceptance criteria are recommended.

The absence of commonly recognized acceptance criteria for these studies has led some laboratories to extreme situations. USP chapter < 1227 > (35) recommends a recovery efficiency of not less than 70% for microbial recovery studies "when the intent is to demonstrate neutralization of antimicrobial properties." The design of this study of antimicrobial neutralization is to take the challenge inoculum, split it into parallel treatment groups, and then treat one with peptone and the other with the product to be tested. The degree of control the technician has over inoculum levels in this design far exceeds that of surface inoculation and recovery after drying. However, the difference in study design has not prevented labs from attempting to apply acceptance criteria of not less than 70% to coupon recovery studies. This is a misapplication of the information found in USP < 1227 > and practitioners are urged to avoid making this mistake.

The validation of recovery efficiency using challenge organisms on a coupon is the most convenient and is widely used. However, it is also the least desirable discussed due to its lack of correlation with the basic nature of the contaminated surfaces seen in the actual sampling event.

ACCURACY/PRECISION OF METHODS

One aspect of microbiological assays that is frequently overlooked is the relationship between the method capabilities and the expected results. This is a particular problem in surface sampling issues for environmental monitoring. While it is extremely tempting to think that we can measure the level of microbial contamination in all areas of the production facility, there are some areas where the observed level of contamination is so low as to fall into the range of "noise" in microbial assays. This does not, however, obviate the need to test in these areas, but we do need to take into account the limitations of our methods when interpreting the data (60). The measurement of the uncertainty in microbiological methods has found its way into the ISO regulations for competency of testing laboratories, which are expected to establish and define the uncertainty of their methods and include this estimate in their reports (61). The units and methods to be used for this estimate are the subject of some discussion (62), as microbiological data offer some challenges to the statistician (63). Microbiological data do not fit a normal distribution and statistics commonly used to create process monitoring controls are not appropriate to this application.

Regulations require, and prudence dictates, measuring the degree of microbial contamination on surfaces in controlled environments, especially those surfaces near open product. However, our methods do not allow for accurate measurement at these levels. This situation has created confusion in the minds of many and has led to a regulatory environment that is not scientifically supportable (64). Let us look at this issue in detail.

Countable Range of CFU on a Plate

This discussion has to start with a consideration of the number of countable colonies on a plate. The lower limit of quantification is set by the nature of the counts, which follow a Poisson distribution (65). The significance of this is that the error of the counts is equal to the square root of the mean. In other words, the relationship between the average estimate of the CFU and the percentage error of the estimates increases dramatically once the CFU/plate drops below 20 (Fig. 2) (7,35). Clearly, any reasonable definition of assay accuracy and precision would require a minimum of 20 CFU/plate for a quantitative assay.

The upper limit of quantification on a plate is a bit more involved. USP $< 1227 >$ gives a general upper limit of 250, but also notes that this is based on the organism's growth characteristics and the surface area of the agar. For example, the currently accepted range of 25 to 250 was "validated" for counting *Escherichia coli* from dairy samples (35), replacing the previously "validated" range of 30 to 300 for the identical application (66). Although demonstrated as appropriate only for *E. coli* from dairy samples, this number has gained wide acceptance for most bacterial colony count applications. However, no one would try to employ that range of CFU on a plate for an assay involving *Aspergillus niger*, which forms large colonies, or for bacterial species which form larger colonies. Likewise, one cannot claim the same upper limit if the surface area of the plate (or membrane filter) is small, as this will encourage occlusion of the colonies, leading to an

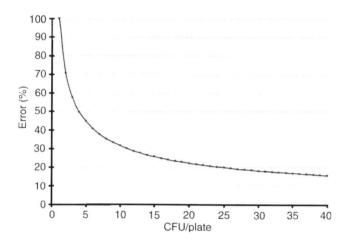

FIGURE 2 Percent error as a function of the estimated CFU per plate. *Abbreviation:* CFU, colony-forming units.

underestimation of CFU. The USP chapter < 1227 > provides a method to determine the upper limit of the counts for a variety of situations.

Here we see a problem—comparing our ability to accurately count CFU and the guidance (Tables 1–3), we have only qualitative measures for the highest controlled rooms. Although the regulations recommend counts less than 10 CFU/plate in several instances, the methods available to us cannot accurately determine those numbers (7,67–70).

Is a Qualitative Evaluation Useful?
The regulatory levels suggested for surface monitoring in the more highly controlled rooms are qualitative at best. Is this really a problem? The first aspect to consider is that the relationship between surface contamination (especially at these levels) and product quality is an assumption. It is a reasonable assumption, so reasonable in fact that several attempts have been made to incorporate this measure into risk assessment models (71–73), but it is an assumption. There are no definitive studies that have shown product contamination as a consequence of a particular level of background microbial load. However, the risk assessment models proposed to date are themselves qualitative in nature, and the imprecision of the microbiological data is not a handicap to their application.

The recognition of the qualitative nature of the data may also encourage new ways of looking at the trending of the information. Several companies have moved away from the arbitrary and inaccurate method of setting alert and action levels by the apparent number of CFU recovered, and have moved to setting alert and action levels based on the frequency of the event in a given period of time (74).

THE ROLE OF MICROBIAL IDENTIFICATION

An understanding of the microbial flora in the manufacturing facility over time is critical. If nothing else, it serves as a means to evaluate the effectiveness of the cleaning protocol for the facility. However, there are a range of identification technologies available to the quality control (QC) microbiology laboratory, and not all applications require the most elaborate methods.

In general, microbial identification methods can be grouped into two categories (75,76):

1. Phenotypic: identification based on the phenotype of the microorganism. These can include standard biochemical methods, the analysis of carbohydrate utilization patterns, and the composition of fatty acid in the microbial cell.
2. Genotypic: identification based on the genotype, or genetic makeup of the cell. These can include DNA fingerprinting by ribotyping, polymerized chain reaction (PCR), or DNA sequencing.

A strong case can be made that phenotypic identification systems are more than adequate for standard trending purposes, although the FDA aseptic processing guidance encourages the use of genotypic methods (75). A real concern is the well-established observation that different identification systems may not provide identical microbial data (77,78). Therefore, performing an investigation with a contaminant identified with one system (perhaps a genotypic system) and including data from a different system is not a valid approach.

A good compromise for many companies is to use phenotypic methods for standard activities, as these are the methods most familiar to the QC microbiology lab. The individual plates are retained until batch release, and then discarded. If needed for an investigation prior to batch release, the retained plates are available for the microbiology laboratory to reidentify the isolates found in the manufacturing facility using the same identification system used for the rest of the investigation.

The identification of the organisms recovered from surfaces and personnel should be identified, at least to the genus level. This information should be included in the environmental-monitoring database and trended along with the rest of the data. As noted above, the isolates (usually as single colony isolate cultures) should be retained at least until the release of the batch is finalized to be available in case of an investigation.

THE POTENTIAL OF RAPID MICROBIOLOGY

The best avenue to real-time release of product is through shortening the time required for microbiological testing (79). This, of course, includes in-process control tests such as surface-monitoring assays. The U.S. FDA has recently issued a guidance document describing the topic of "process analytical technology," designed to encourage the use of in-process controls to increase product quality through advances in technology (80). This approach has encouraged some very thoughtful evaluations. Korczynski developed an integrated approach to product quality in a well-reasoned and comprehensive review (81). He argued that PAT is one of several quality initiatives [including Hazard Analysis Critical Control Points (HACCP), concurrent validation, and parametric release] with the potential to dramatically improve the final product quality through control of the process. This approach, he argued, could result in greatly reducing the number of number of release tests, although it could not remove the need for sterility testing at present.

Several authors have recently described the potential for rapid microbiological methods in in-process testing. Moldenhauer (82), Cundell (83), Sutton (84), and

Miller (85) provide overviews of the regulatory approaches and validation concerns associated with the implementation of the different methods, but it should also be noted here that most of the methods used for surface monitoring are not generally part of a regulatory submission. The test methods for surface monitoring (RODAC and swabs) can be adapted for a rapid test (86) and would provide real advantages to the company in terms of immediate feedback on the state of control of the facility. Among these are ATP bioluminescence (87), autofluorescence (88), flow cytometry (89), solid-phase cytometry (90), PCR (45,91), and others.

There are many opportunities for the use of rapid microbiological methods in the monitoring of solid surfaces as well as other applications in the environmental-monitoring program. These have the potential to dramatically decrease the amount of time required for results to be reported, and potential increase the usefulness of the data. The interested reader is referred to the review articles referenced above for more information on these methods.

CONCLUSIONS

Surface monitoring is a critical component to the demonstration of the state of control of the manufacturing environment, but it cannot be linked to finished product quality at the present time. There are several different methods used to monitor surfaces, each of them has its own particular strengths and weaknesses.

The validation or qualification of surface-monitoring methods is confounded by technical difficulties. One common method is to inoculate the surface with a controlled inoculum and calculate recovery from the inoculum level. This suffers from issues with desiccation and the concern that this results in an artificial situation. A second method utilizes natural bioburden with repetitive sampling. This method of validation can be analyzed either by linear regression or by total recovery.

The data in itself is a concern, as frequently regulatory documents recommend levels below the ability of the methods to accurately measure. Suggestions are provided on how to design alert and action levels that reflect this limitation.

The reliance on standard microbiological methods ensures that the in-process surface-monitoring data will not be available for several days. The use of rapid microbiological alternative methods can be justified as process improvements, allowing close to real-time microbiological control data on the manufacturing process.

REFERENCES

1. Agalloco J et al. Aseptic processing: a review of current industry practice. Pharm Technol Oct 2004; 126–150.
2. Akers JE. Environmental monitoring and control: proposed standards, current practices. PDA J Pharm Sci Technol 1997; 51:36–47.
3. Hertroys R et al. Moving towards a (microbiological) environmental monitoring program that can be used to release aseptically produced pharmaceuticals: a hypothesis, a practical programme and some results. PDA J Pharm Sci Technol 1997; 51:52–59.
4. Lindsay J. Experience in Media Fills at PDA TRI, Poster Presentation at PDA Spring 2002 Meeting, 2002.
5. FDA. Guidance for industry: sterile drug products produced by aseptic processing—current good manufacturing practice, 2004.
6. Cundell AM. Microbial testing in support of aseptic processing. Pharm Technol 2004; 28(6):58–66.
7. Hussong D, Madsen RE. Analysis of environmental microbiology data from cleanroom samples. Pharm Technol 2004 (Aseptic Proc Issue):10–15.
8. Hyde WA. Origin of bacteria in the clean room and their growth requirements. PDA J Pharm Sci Technol 1998; 52(4):154–158.
9. PIC/S. PI 014-1: Recommendation on isolators used for aseptic processing and sterility testing, 2002.
10. PIC/S. PI-006-2: Recommendations on validation master plan, installation and operational qualification, non-sterile process validation, cleaning validation, 2004.
11. Tidswell E. Risk-based approaches facilitate expedient validations for control of microorganisms during equipment cleaning and hold. Am Pharm Rev 2005; 8:28–33.
12. LeBlanc DA. Equipment cleaning validation: microbial control issues. J Validation Technol 2002; 8:40–46.
13. Sutton SVW. Disinfectant rotation—a microbiologist's view. Control Environ 2005; 8(7):9–14.
14. Sartain EK. Designing a cleanroom disinfectant program to meet production requirements and regulatory expectations. A2C2 2004; 7(12):21–24.
15. PDA. PDA Tech Report #13: fundamentals of a microbiological environmental monitoring program. PDA J Parenter Sci Technol 1990; 44:S3–S16.
16. USP < 1116 >. Microbiological control and monitoring environments used for the manufacture of healthcare products. Pharm Forum 2005; 31(2):524–549.
17. PDA. Tech Report #13 (Revised): fundamentals of an environmental monitoring program. PDA J Pharm Sci Technol 2001; 55:1–36.
18. Cowell ND, Morisetti MD. Microbiological techniques—some statistical aspects. J Sci Food Agric 1969; 20:573–579.
19. Stearman RL. Statistical concepts in microbiology. Bacteriol Rev 1955; 19:160–215.
20. Cundell A et al. Statistical analysis of environmental monitoring data: does a worst case time for monitoring clean rooms exist? PDA J Pharm Sci Technol 1998; 52(6):326–330.
21. Wilson J. Setting alert/action limits for environmental monitoring programs. PDA J Pharm Sci Technol 1997; 51:161–162.
22. Westney R. Strategies for managing environmental monitoring investigations. Am Pharm Rev 2005; 8(4):18–31.
23. Akers JE, Agalloco JP. Recent inspectional trends: are regulatory requirements for sterite products becoming scientifically undoable or impractical? PDAJ pharm Sci Technol 2002; 56(4):179–182.

24. Baldock JD. Microbiological monitoring of the food plant: methods to assess bacterial contamination on surfaces. J Milk Food Technol 1974; 37(7):1974.
25. PDA. PDA Tech Report #24: current practices in the validation of aseptic processing—1996. PDA J Pharm Sci Technol 1997; 51(2).
26. PDA. PDA Tech Report #36: Current practices in the validation of aseptic processing—2001. PDA J Pharm Sci Technol 2002; 56(3).
27. Niskanen A, Pohja MS. Comparative studies on the sampling and investigation of microbial contamination of surfaces by the contact plate and swab methods. J Appl Bacteriol 1977; 42:53–63.
28. Hall LB, Hartnett MJ. Measurement of the bacterial contamination on surfaces. Pub Health Report 1964; 79:1021–1024.
29. Bruch M. Improved method for pouring RODAC plates. Appl Microbiol 1968; 16(9):1427–1428.
30. Rohde PA. A new culture plate: its applications. PDA Bull Parent Drug Assoc 1963; 17(1):11–13.
31. Keenan KM et al. Some statistical problems in the standardization of a method for sampling surfaces for microbiological contamination. Hosp Lab Serv 1965; 2:208–215.
32. Dey BP. Comparison of Dey and Engley (D/E) neutralizing medium to letheen medium and standard methods medium for recovery of *Staphylococcus aureus* from sanitized surfaces. J Ind Microbiol 1995; 14:21–25.
33. Schiemann DA. Evaluation of neutralizers in RODAC media for microbial recovery from disinfected floors. J Environ Health 1976; 38(6):401–404.
34. Tomasiewicz DM et al. The most suitable number of colonies on plates for counting. J Food Prot 1980; 43(4):282–286.
35. USP < 1227 >. Validation of microbial recovery from pharmacopeial articles. In: USP 29 United States Pharmacopeial Convention, Washington, DC, 2006:3053–3055.
36. Speck ML, Black LA. Effectiveness of cotton-swab methods in bacteriological examination of paper ice cream containers. Food Res 1937; 2:559–566.
37. Richard J. Observations on the value of a swab technique for determining the bacteriological state of milking equipment surfaces. J Appl Bacteriol 1980; 49:19–27.
38. Rose L et al. Swab materials and *Bacillus anthracis* spore recovery from nonporous surfaces. Emerg Infect Dis 2004; 10(6):1023–1029.
39. Lemmen S et al. Comparison of two sampling methods for the detection of gram-positive and gram-negative bacteria in the environment: moistened swabs versus RODAC plates. Int J Hyg Environ Health 2001; 203:245–248.
40. Cate L. A note on a simple and rapid method of bacteriological sampling by means of agar sausages. J Appl Bacteriol 1965; 28(2):221–223.
41. Angelotti R, Foter MJ. A direct surface agar plate laboratory method for quantitatively detecting bacterial contamination on nonporous surfaces. Am J Public Health Sep 1957; 170–174.
42. Pitzurra M et al. A new method to study the microbial contamination of surfaces. Hyg Med 1997; 22:77–92.
43. Poletti L et al. Comparative efficiency of nitrocellulose membranes versus RODAC plates in microbial sampling on surfaces. J Hosp Infect 1999; 41:195–201.
44. Craythorn J et al. Membrane filter contact technique for bacteriological sampling of moist surfaces. J Clin Microbiol 1980; 12(2):250–255.
45. Buttner MP et al. Evaluation of the Biological Sampling Kit (BiSKit) for large-area surface sampling. Appl Environ Microbiol 2004; 70(12):7040–7045.
46. Clark DS. Method of estimating the bacterial population on surfaces. Can J Microbiol 1965; 11:407–413.

47. Williamson P et al. A new method for the quantitative investigation of cutaneous bacteria. J Invest Derm 1965; 45(6):498–503.
48. Salo S et al. Validation of the microbiological methods hygicult dipslide, contact plate, and swabbing in surface hygiene control: a nordic collaborative study. J AOAC Int 2000; 83(6):1357–1365.
49. Moldenhauer J. Surface monitoring. In: Moldenhauer J, ed. Environmental Monitoring: A Comprehensive Handbook. River Grove: DHI Publishers, 2005:339–356.
50. ISO. EN 1174–1 Sterilization of medical devices—estimation of the population of micro organisms on product—Part I, 1996.
51. ISO. ISO 11737–1 Sterilization of medical devices—microbiological methods—Part 1: Estimation of population of microorganisms on products, 1995.
52. Favero MS et al. Microbiological sampling of surfaces. J Appl Bacteriol 1968; 31:336–343.
53. Bakker DP et al. Bacterial strains isolated from different niches can exhibit different patterns of adhesion to substrata. Appl Environ Microbiol 2004; 70(6):3758–3760.
54. Douglas J. Recovery of known numbers of micro-organisms from surfaces by swabbing. Lab Pract 1968; 17(12):1336–1337.
55. Potts M. Desiccation tolerance of prokaryotes. Microbiol Rev 1994; 58(4):755–805.
56. Whyte W. Methods for calculating the efficiency of bacterial surface sampling techniques. J Hosp Infect 1989; 13:33–41.
57. Yamayoshi T et al. Surface sampling using a single swab method. J Hosp Infect 1984; 5:386–390.
58. Eginton PJ. Quantification of the ease of removal of bacteria from surfaces. J Indust Microbiol 1995; 15:305–310.
59. PDA. PDA Technical Report #21: Bioburden recovery validation. PDA J Parent Sci Technol 1990; 44(6):324–331.
60. Akers J, Moore C. The need for pragmatism. A2C2 Jan 1998; 23–30.
61. ISO. ISO/IEC 17025 General requirements for the competence of testing and calibration laboratories, 1999.
62. Forster LI. Measurement uncertainty in microbiology. J AOAC Int 2003; 86:1089–1094.
63. Ilstrup D. Statistical methods in microbiology. Clin Microbiol Rev 1990; 3:219–226.
64. Akers JE. Science based aseptic processing. PDA J Pharm Sci Technol 2002; 56(6):283–290.
65. Eisenhart C, Perry W. Statistical methods and control in bacteriology. Bacteriol Rev 1943; 7:57–137.
66. Breed R, Dotterrer WD. The number of colonies allowable on satisfactory agar plates. J Bacteriol 1916; 1:321–331.
67. Wilson J. Environmental monitoring: misconceptions and misapplications. PDA J Pharm Sci Technol 2001; 55:185–190.
68. Akers JE, Agalloco J. Environmental monitoring: myths and misapplications. PDA J Pharm Sci Technol 2001; 55:176–184.
69. Akers JE, Agalloco JP. Aseptic processing, elephants, blind men and sterility. PDA J Pharm Sci Technol 2002; 56:231–234.
70. Hussong D, Mello R. Alternative microbiology methods and pharmaceutical quality control. Am Pharm Rev 2006; 9(1):62–68.
71. Eaton T. Microbial risk assessment for aseptically prepared products. Am Pharm Rev 2005; 8:46–51.
72. Eaton T. Microbial risk assessments for pharmaceutical products. Cleanroom Monitor S2C2 2005; 52:1–12.

73. Akers J, Agalloco J. Risk analysis for aseptic processing: the Akers–Agalloco method. Pharm Technol 2005; 29:74–88.
74. Caputo RA, Huffman A. Environmental monitoring: data trending using a frequency model. PDA J Pharm Sci Technol 2004; 58:254–260.
75. Sutton SVW, Cundell AM. Microbial identification in the pharmaceutical industry. Pharm Forum 2004; 30(5):1884–1894.
76. Cundell AM. Microbial identification strategies in the pharmaceutical industry. PDA J Pharm Sci Technol 2006; 60(2):111–123.
77. Tang Y et al. Comparison of phenotypic and genotypic techniques for identification of unusual aerobic pathogenic gram-negative bacilli. J Clin Microbiol 1998; 36(12):3674–3679.
78. Stager CE, Davis JR. Automated systems for identification of microorganisms. Clin Microbiol Rev 1992; 5(3):302–327.
79. Singer DC, Cundell AM. The role of rapid microbiological methods within the process analytical technology initiative. Pharm Forum 2003; 29(6):2109–2113.
80. FDA. Guidance for industry: Process analytical technology—a framework for innovative pharmaceutical development, manufacturing, and quality assurance, 2004.
81. Korczynski MS. The integration of process analytical technologies, concurrent validation, and parametric release programs in aseptic processing. PDA J Pharm Sci Technol 2004; 58(4):181–191.
82. Moldenhauer J. An overview of rapid microbiology methods. Pharm Form Quality Jun/Jul 2004; 61–64.
83. Cundell AM. Opportunities for rapid microbial methods. Eur Pharm Rev 2006; 1:64–70.
84. Sutton SVW. Validation of alternative microbiology methods for product testing: Quantitative and qualitative assays. Pharm Technol 2005; 29(4):118–122.
85. Miller MJ. Rapid Microbiological methods and FDA's initiatives for pharmaceutical cGMP's for the 21st century, PAT and sterile drug products produced by aseptic processing. Am Pharm Rev 2005; 8(1):104–107.
86. Sutton SV. Opportunities for the pharmaceutical industry. In: Miller M, ed. Encyclopedia of Rapid Microbiological Methods. Vol. 1. Washington, DC: DHI Publications, 2005:123–156.
87. Buttner M et al. Enhanced detection of surface-associated bacteria in indoor environments by quantitative PCR. Appl Environ Microbiol 2001; 67(6):2564–2570.
88. Bolotin C. Instantaneous microbial detection. Control Environ 2005; 8(12):10–15.
89. Veal DA et al. Florescence staining and flow cytometry for monitoring microbial cells. J Immunol Meth 2000; 243:191–210.
90. Brailsford M. Making the switch to real-time microbiological process control. Manuf Chem 1997; 35–36.
91. Nadkarni M. Determination of bacterial load by real-time PCR using a broad-range (universal) probe and primers set. Microbiology 2002; 148:257–266.

6 Process Simulations (Media Fills)

Anne Marie Dixon

6   Process Simulations (Media Fills)

Anne Marie Dixon

Cleanroom Management Associates, Inc., Carson City, Nevada, U.S.A.

BACKGROUND

Sterile pharmaceuticals are either by aseptic processing techniques or by terminal sterilization methods. In aseptic processing, the drug product, container, and enclosure are presterilized and the filling operations are performed in high quality environments, traditionally called cleanrooms. Aseptic processing can provide products with a high degree of sterility assurance when they are carried out under stringent aseptic processing conditions with well-defined standards. In the 1960s and 1970s, the aseptic processing methods, even when performed under optimal conditions, could only be validated to ensure that the contamination rate is no greater than one contaminated unit per thousand (10^{-3}) filled. Today, processing technologies have emerged and are capable of minimizing or eliminating human intervention with proper techniques, proper gowning, effective sanitization of surfaces, and sterile materials.

The word "validation" first appeared in print in the 1978 revision to the current good manufacturing practices regulations (cGMPs) (1). Section 211.113 ("Control of Microbiological Contamination") of the cGMP requires the establishment of, and adherence to, "appropriate written procedures designed to prevent microbial contamination of drug products purporting to be sterile. Such procedures must include validation of any sterilization process" (2).

In 1987, Food and Drug Administration (FDA) published a guideline that addressed acceptable practices and procedures for the preparation of drug products by aseptic processing according to the cGMP regulations (3). Validation was defined in this document as "...establishing documented evidence which provides a high degree of assurance that a specific process will consistently produce product meeting its predetermined specifications and quality attributed" (3).

Two issues must be considered in the validation of any aseptic process. First, the drug substance itself and all the necessary components for formulation and filling need to be processed using procedures and equipment that have been validated to assure sterility. Second, the aseptic assembly process, i.e., the filling operation, needs to be validated separately to demonstrate that the process of assembly does not compromise the sterility of individual components and finished product. One of the most difficult and important tasks in pharmaceutical production is that of an aseptic process validation. The requirement for validation forced the industry to begin thinking carefully about how to formally qualify facilities and institute appropriate controls for aseptic processing.

"The aseptic process simulation is widely used for the validation of aseptic processing. The test substitutes sterile microbiological growth medium for sterile products and so is referred to as media fill" (4). During a media fill, the exposure to operators, mechanics, samplers, interventions, components, and the filling environment (air cleanliness) all affect the nutrient sterile medium's chances of becoming contaminated. If growth is observed in a media fill, it is assumed that the process is not in control, and that there is a chance that routine production is incapable of producing a sterile drug product.

FDA's "Aseptic Processing Guideline" in 1987 describes a media fill as "an" acceptable method of validating aseptic manufacturing, not as "the only" acceptable method. However, by the 1990s, both the FDA and the EU GMPs included requirements for media fills in support of aseptic processes. Because of the sensitivity of the microbiological growth medium to overt contamination, media fills are now the generally accepted approach for validating the adequacy of protection from microbial contamination afforded by the aseptic filling process as well as for identifying potential weaknesses in the operation that might contribute to contamination of the drug product.

In addition to demonstrating that the aseptic fill/finish process is capable of producing a sterile drug product, process simulations are used to qualify or certify aseptic processing personnel (including operators, mechanics, and samplers), validate a new facility, validate significant changes to a filling record, and validate new filling line equipment. Each of these aspects of the media fill is now an expectation of current GMPs.

CONTAMINATION SOURCES

People

Cleanroom environments containing people are never sterile. Maintaining safe product conditions throughout the processing is extremely important. It is recognized throughout the industry that the final product testing is inadequate to totally assure the sterility of any aseptically filled product (5). Microbial contamination for sterile products manufactured by aseptic process is mainly caused by human intervention. Cleanroom operators generate millions of particles with every movement. Every employee who enters an aseptic area must have successfully completed training and qualifications in gowning, cleanroom disciplines, basic microbiology, and aseptic techniques prior to entrance. Particles can and do migrate through the cleanroom apparel. Complete barrier gowning is required—full hood, coverall, facemask, protective goggles, gloves, and boots. If a garment does not seal at the neck or around the eye area, or is oversized, particulates from the head and sleeve will vent into the cleanroom environment above the working level because of the bellows effect.

Personnel-associated product contamination may occur by direct or indirect routes. Touching a sterile instrument with a nonsterile gloved hand, for example, can result in direct contamination. In contrast, an indirect contamination is caused by poor adherence to procedures intended to minimize contamination load and dispersal throughout the cleanroom. For example, personnel can create turbulence by rapid movements, increasing the chance of indirect contamination. Poor gowning techniques, failure to follow written procedures, and failure to minimize the frequency of entrances and exits could also establish the potential for indirect contamination risk.

The quality of filling under aseptic conditions will vary with the training, experience, motivation, and operational familiarity of each operator to the machine, equipment, cleanroom, and the fatigue of the operator. In general, a media fill should simulate the worst-case conditions that might exist during normal operations. It should challenge the operators to the same extent that would be expected during the lengthiest, most complex production run.

There is a minimum requirement to involve individuals in at least one process simulation (operators, mechanics, and quality assurance personnel) on an annual basis. However, in order to maintain their aseptic awareness and validation status, it makes good sense to incorporate as many people as possible in each process simulation trial.

Equipment

Unvalidated sterilization/depyrogenation/sanitization cycles for product contact equipment or components (vials/stoppers) can result in a lack of assurance sterility or an endotoxin contamination event. Likewise, inadequate cleaning of product contact surfaces prior to sterilization could result in product carryover and crosscontamination.

Room Environment

Proper cleanroom conditions are demonstrated by the proper qualification of heating, ventilation and air conditioning (HVAC) systems, utility systems (including water), cleaning and sanitization procedures, proper gowning procedures, and limiting access only to trained/qualified people.

Patched, poor, or uncertified high-efficiency particulate air (HEPA) filters, inadequate air change rates, loss of pressurization, and lack of procedures to come back into production after a loss of pressurization can adversely affect the aseptic manufacturing environment.

All utilities that come into contact with sterile components or sterile product must be designed to provide assurance of sterility. Water for injection (WFI) systems must undergo a stringent qualification process to demonstrate that they are capable of consistently delivering high quality water. Gasses, particularly those that come into contact with product as overlays or vessel purges, must be filtered at the point of use (6).

All cleanroom surfaces including walls, ceilings, benches, floors, doors, phones, intercoms, vents, and filling equipment must be cleaned and sanitized using validated procedures. Validation of cleaning and sanitization includes choice of sanitizers, testing of sanitizers to demonstrate efficacy both in vitro and in situ, testing of product contact surfaces for residuals, rotation of disinfectants/sanitizers as needed, the cleaning method itself (mops, wipes), and the proper training of cleaning personnel.

Environmental Monitoring

Environmental monitoring, if not performed correctly, can be a source of contamination. Training must include demonstration of aseptic technique, the ability to completely remove any contact plate residuals, an understanding of laminarity, and how to perform monitoring without disturbing operators or equipment.

A poorly conceived environmental monitoring program can be detrimental to an aseptic process in that inappropriate sampling locations and frequencies or lack of data analysis will result in a failure to recognize adverse trends in the environmental quality.

THE PROCESS OF DEVISING, EXECUTING, AND ASSESSING MEDIA FILLS

Establishment of a Program

The first step in establishing a media fill program is the drafting of a broad policy, a document that may be in the form of a memo, master plan, policy statement, standard operating procedure, or validation protocol. This policy document should define the purpose of the program, a risk analysis, the frequency of routine revalidation, and nonroutine reasons for revalidation. A crossfunctional group that includes manufacturing, validation, and quality should draft the document. The roles and responsibilities of each function or group such as the microbiologist, engineers, the quality experts, operational staff, and management should be defined.

A media fill program should incorporate the contamination risk factors that occur on a production line and accurately assess the state of process control. The risks to be included are:

- People
- Equipment
- Components
- Facility and utilities

A recommended media fill program incorporates the contamination risk factors that occur on a production line and accurately assesses the state of process control. Media fill studies should simulate aseptic manufacturing process operations as closely as possible, incorporating a worst-case approach. The media fill program should address the applicable issues as such:

1. Equipment

    - Factors associated with the longest permitted run on the processing line
    - Number and type of normal interventions, e.g., maintenance, stoppages, and equipment adjustments
    - Line speed and configuration
    - Lyophilization where applicable
    - Aseptic assembly of equipment (e.g., startup)

2. Personnel

    - Number of personnel and their activities
    - Shift changes, breaks, and gown changes
    - Operator fatigue

3. Operations

    - Number of aseptic additions
    - Number and type of aseptic equipment disconnect and connections
    - Aseptic sample of collection
    - Manual weight checks
    - Container closure system
    - Specific provisions for aseptic processing-related standard operating procedures

Media fills should never be used to justify an unacceptable practice. A solid media fill program is the key to acceptable manufacturing success and it can be assured by good planning and operational staff input.

Protocol Preparation

The detailed planning is the second step of this program and it should include the identification of the risk variables in defining the worst case. Once the process has been clearly defined, the media fill or appropriate standard operating procedure or validation protocol can be written. A protocol in the form of a batch record must be prepared for each run on each line. This document should include, but is not limited to, the following:

- Identification of the process (lyo, aseptic fill in preparation for TS, powder fill, liquid fill)
- Identification of the room
- Identification of the filling line and equipment
- Type of container/closure to be used
- Line speed
- Number of units to be filled
- Number and type of interventions
- Number of personnel to participate
- Type of media to be used
- Volume of medium to be filled into the containers
- Incubator identification and incubation time and temperature
- Environmental monitoring
- Copy of the batch record to be used
- Acceptance criteria for the test
- Description of documentation record for the final report
- Box or tray number of positive units
- Growth support testing requirements and result
- Rationale for worst-case "parameters" chosen
- Summation of the data from the batch record environmental monitoring samples based upon this information, a conclusion is formulated regarding the acceptability of the manufacturing process and the facility
- Aseptic set up and assembly of sterile equipment

All personnel who enter the aseptic processing area, including technicians and maintenance personnel, should participate in a media fill at least once per year as part of the operator qualification process.

Process Parameters

Production Batch Size/Media Fill
The duration and size of the fill must be reflective of the actual product being manufactured. The duration of the run should be sufficient to ensure that the necessary number of units and activities are included. A minimum number of 5000 filled containers are specified in the FDA aseptic product manufacturing guidelines on 30 September 2004. A generally accepted media fill size is from 5000 to 10,000 units. A hold time for the bulk media should be established for each media fill. Initially, the hold time should mimic the production hold times.

The speed and a line configuration of the filling process are parameters that are highly dependent on the individual line being challenged. In many situations, the "worst case" is the speed that provides for the greatest exposure of media to environmental conditions, i.e., the slowest speed and the largest vial neck opening. However, many production lines that fill very small vials at fast speeds can create the greatest number of jammed containers, misfilled product, or manual interventions. It is advisable to use a risk assessment to determine the most critical parameters.

Using "industry standard definitions" of worst-case scenarios is not a substitute for a thorough understanding of the process being validated. After an evaluation of the process and the batch parameters, the fill protocol must represent the most difficult manufacturing period.

A media filled batch record must be prepared. Media filled documents are most useful as process validation and training exercises when the document is identical as close as possible to the actual manufacturing batch. The batch record documenting production conditions and simulated activity should be prepared for each media filled line. The same vigilance that is used for routine production must be observed in both media fill and routine production runs. One addition to the batch record that has proved to be a useful tool is a typical table that lists where real or simulated line jams are cleared, spills cleared, or rejected vials are removed from the line. This table will reflect that a given action is supported by the media fill and can also serve as a reminder to the operators what interventions need to be performed.

When the aseptic filling process is performed manually or the practice of any other extensive manual manipulations, the duration of the process simulation should generally be no less than the length of the actual manufacturing process to best simulate contamination risks as posed by the operator. For operations with production sizes under 5000, the number of media vials should be equal to the maximum batch size made on a processing line. For very small batch sizes, which are common in clinical practices and in some biological practices, the volume should be equal to that of the production or the clinical trial run. This is to simulate a day's worth of filling.

Interventions

It is expected that a predetermined list of all permitted interventions be maintained and incorporated into the process simulation on a periodic basis. Typical interventions should be performed during each process simulation. Atypical intervention should be performed at least once per year. Process simulation tests must include all normal activities that occur during an aseptic filling process in order to substantiate the acceptability of those practices and routine operation. Routine interventions include:

- Aseptic assembly of the equipment
- Bulk connection and startup of the line
- Initial weight and/or volume checks
- Periodic weight and/or volume checks
- Addition of components
- Operator breaks
- Product sampling
- Filter integrity testing
- Environmental monitoring
- Any other activity that is part of a normal operational process

It is possible that a nonplanned intervention may be necessary to correct for container breakage and fluid leakage jams which may occur during the process simulation. In addition to these, the following are examples of nonroutine activities:

- Stopper jam
- Broken containers
- Product spills
- Adjustments of fill head assemblies

■ Equipment change-out
■ Removal of components
■ Any other malfunction that could require a manual adjustment

The interventions should be reviewed and discussed in detail in order to determine those that must be included in each media fill. Operators should be trained in the execution of these interventions (7). Proper documentation is required for all interventions in the batch record. The documentation should include the time the event occurred and the identification of the event.

Large Batch Size

For these types of processes where high-speed fillers are commonplace, a minimum of 5000 units should be filled in order to accommodate the number of interventions normally used in production. There are a number of ways to accomplish this in order to achieve all the interventions and show both the stress of the cleanroom and the fatigue of the operator. In order to simulate specific time duration, it should be ensured that media units are filled at the beginning, middle, and end of a specific time duration. Media should also be filled to simulate change-out of personnel at break times. Consider the following example:

1. Fill 3000 units with medium, switch to sterile WFI for an extended period of time; fill an additional 3000 units with medium. Alternate WFI with medium over the course of the day in order to show the stress of the fill line as well as the stress of the operator. (Note of caution: it is difficult to reconcile the total media quantity, as residual in the line will cross into the WFI units. These units will also require incubation. However, if the growth medium gets diluted out to the point where it is not a factor, and the diluted media is not validated for growth promotion, it may be difficult to determine if there is a failure or an invalid growth occurrence.)
2. Fill 3000 with medium, run glass and stoppers without any liquid being added for an extended period of time, and then fill an additional 3000 units of medium throughout the day. There is a current concern that switching from medium to WFI will allow for bleed-over into the vials. Because the vials are now deluded, should the vials be incubated? What would the results mean? How these vials are to be handled? Therefore, it is the opinion of the author that running the line between media vials, without any liquid, does simulate the fill line being run, the stress of the cleanroom, and potential stress of the operator.

Filling Speed

In general, a fill speed, used for any container, should be set at the low end of the filling range for the size container. If a higher speed results in the potential for greater interventions, then the speed should be considered when selecting process simulation test parameters in the validation protocol.

The duration of the run should be sufficient to cover all manipulations that are normally performed in actual manufacturing. The number of test units should reflect the worst-case exposure time at filling rates that are equivalent to or slower than actual production filling speeds.

Lyophilized Filled Product

Most lyophilized products are aseptically filled solutions that are transferred to a sterile lyophilization chamber after filling. It is an industry practice to simulate lyophilization as part of the media or process simulation protocol. Containers are filled with medium and stoppers are partially inserted into the necks. The containers are manually or robotically transported and loaded into the lyophilizer. A full or partial vacuum is drawn on the chamber at ambient temperature and maintained for the duration of a normal lyophilization process. The chamber is then vented and the stoppers are seated within the chamber. The stoppered units are removed from the aseptic area and sealed and transported for incubation. The advantage of this type of simulation is that the medium is not frozen. Therefore, there are fewer concerns with regard to microbial survival.

However, this type of process has some disadvantages. The amount of time required to perform the entire lyophilization cycle is extensive. The vacuum must not be so low as to permit the medium and the container to boil out.

A compromise should be considered. There is the ability to do a simulated load with a shortened time. These containers are filled and stoppers are partially inserted into the necks. The units are manually or robotically loaded into the lyophilizer, partial vacuum is drawn, and is held for a predetermined time. The chamber is then vented and the stoppers are seated within the chamber. These units are returned for aseptic processing area, sealed, and transported for incubation. The disadvantage of this is that the shortened time exposure may not simulate the actual lyophilization process duration adequately and the potential risk of contamination during the normal process cycle time.

Anaerobic Conditions

Manufacturers that fill a number of aerobically processed products are advised to perform a periodic process simulation using appropriate anaerobic medium, e.g., alternate fluid thioglycollate without agar. The use of an inert gas and anaerobic medium (e.g., alternate fluid thioglycollate medium) would be appropriate when the presence of anaerobic organisms has been confirmed either during the environmental monitoring or more likely during sterility product testing.

In addition to using the thioglycollate medium, manufacturers are also advised to perform an aerobic fill using a growth medium such as soybean casein digest, with a compressed air overlay. This will simulate the turbulence in the product container and allow for environmental data for aerobic organisms.

Regardless of the fill type, one should address anaerobes during media fills— especially facultative anaerobes from personnel.

Media Growth Promotion

In general, a microbial growth medium such as soybean casein digest medium should be used. This media selected should be demonstrated to promote growth of United States Pharmacopoeia (USP) <71> indicated organisms as well as representative isolates identified from environmental monitoring, personal monitoring, and positive sterility test results.

Positive control units should be inoculated with a less than 100 colony-forming units challenge and incubated. For those instances in which growth promotion testing fails, the origin of any contamination found during the simulation should be nevertheless investigated and the media fill should be promptly repeated. Growth promotion of media in the units is most meaningful if they are performed at the same time as the possible contamination of an aseptically filled product, i.e., a randomly selected unit in parallel with the incubation of the media fill. It is recommended to perform a growth promotion at the beginning and at the end (i.e., incubated vials) to demonstrate that the incubation conditions were not detrimental to the growth of organisms.

Growth promotion at the end of the incubation may not detect any interaction between the contaminants and the containers that may mask gross inhibition. Testing of the final media may prove useful if the media fill has failed. However, if the residual media fails and the media fill passes, the results of the media fill must stand. The inability of incubated units to demonstrate growth on the growth promotion does not invalidate the run. However, there needs to be an investigation. If the growth promotion is a type of "system suitability," it is important to understand what this type of failure would indicate.

Environmental Conditions

These are controversial factors in media fill scenarios. While operations staff acknowledges that environmental conditions may have a significant impact on sterility assurance, cleanroom managers are rightfully against including any intentional falsification of environmental control.

The best middle ground may be to conduct media fills during times that reflect full range of environmental variation, such as before and after maintenance shutdowns as well as mid-production times, seasonal variation that effect humidity, or stressing the cleanability of the cleanroom.

It should be stated that altering the operational conditions of a cleanroom outside the basis of design could have a significant impact on the cleanroom, HVAC system, and HEPA filtration systems. Generally, if a product fill would be aborted, then a media fill is also aborted.

Filled Volume

This volume should be sufficient to assess potential microbial contamination and to ensure the complete contact of all sterile surfaces inside the container when inverted.

Regardless of the actual fill volume selected, the process simulation test should include a fill weight adjustment using methods identical to those employed during production.

Incubation

The conditions suitable for recovery of bioburden and environmental monitoring isolates should be not less than 14 days at a temperature between 20°C and 35°C. The temperature chosen should be based upon the ability to recover microorganisms normally found environmentally or in the product bioburden.

Many firms prefer a two-temperature incubation schedule to incubate at 20°C to 25°C for a minimum of seven days followed by incubation at a higher temperature range, which is not to exceed 35°C for a total minimum incubation time of 14 days.

It is a generally accepted practice that prior to incubation, the containers are inverted or otherwise manipulated to ensure that all the surfaces, including the internal surface of the closure, are thoroughly wetted by the media. These containers should not be completely filled with media in order to provide sufficient oxygen for the growth of obligate aerobes.

The concept of process simulation is to assess the potential contamination in units that are representative of normal production cycles. The requirement to incubate and include the evaluation of procedurally excluded units, those used for process testing or interventions (when the removal of such units is reproducible and clearly documented in the routine production), does not assess the potential of the production for nonsterile units. The inclusion of procedurally excluded units presents an artificially stringent measure of the capability of an aseptic process. However, removing units that under normal filling would not be removed is totally unacceptable. There must be a control mechanism for exclusion and a full accountability of these units.

Many firms perform an inspection of units leaving the filling area for broken, noticeably cracked, or without stoppers or crimps. All such units, if discarded, must be recorded with a description of the fault.

Reconciliation requirements for process simulation units should be equivalent to the requirement for a production size run. A 100% reconciliation accountability of all units filled should be the target.

Two reconciliations must be performed prior to incubation. The first reconciliation is of the total number of units filled. Generally, there are three categories of containers:

1. Group I: marketable product and vials with cosmetic defects from post fill inspection operations
2. Group II: intervention—units removed
3. Group III: defects—cracks, no stoppers, leaks

All containers in Group I must be incubated. No containers can be discarded.

The second reconciliation is for the media. Accountability must be performed for the total bulk media. As an example, assume 1000 L of media has been prepared, then:

1000L – total volume

– 600L – filled

– 375L – residual in the bulk tank

 – 5L – surge tank residual

 – 20L – lines, filters, assemblies, waste, purge

 = TOTALLY RECONCILED BULK

Generally, these two reconciliations are included in the batch record.

Acceptance Criteria

Equipment failures, environmental excursions, and staff shortages can have a dramatic impact on the media fill, just as they do on routine production. It is essential that all staff members be trained to report deviations from the plan so a decision may be made immediately to keep or discard the vials.

The definition of an accepted media fill is one of the most critical variations between regulatory agencies. The FDA guidance document on 30 September 2004 specifies that growth in a single vial must be thoroughly investigated and will result in failure for small fill quantities. ISO guidelines are more lenient relying on the statistical analysis of 0.1% contamination with a 95% confidence level. However, the expectation is no contamination regardless of the lot size. A research article (8) indicated that the existing criteria, such as "less than 0.1%," "less than 0.05%," and less than two positives, are not appropriate to assure the integrity of processes and sometimes lead to erroneous results.

However, persistent low levels of contaminated vials should be taken as an indication of a manufacturing problem, even if the media fill passed formal acceptance criteria. Any positive unit indicates a potential problem regardless of the run size. All positives of media and environmental should be identified to genus and species. These identified positives should be compared to previous environmental and personnel isolates. All positives should result in a thorough, documented, investigation. If the positives are indicative of an unacceptable practice, e.g., a particular type of intervention, the procedure must be analyzed, and SOPs must be written and implemented after proper training. It is advisable that water fill training be performed prior to the rerun of a media fill to ensure that the practices are acceptable.

Consecutive acceptable media fill simulations are required to initially validate a new process. After the initial testing, regular validation is required. In the United States, a media fill must be repeated at six-month intervals. Other regulatory jurisdictions require a minimum of four media fills per year. Specific requirements for each jurisdiction should be also reviewed periodically.

Generally, three consecutive successful process simulation tests are performed when qualifying a new facility or filling line or validating a process. Prior to the release of a new facility, filling line, or process for production use, acceptable results from these consecutive tests should be achieved to demonstrate the reproducibility of the process. It is current industry standard that media fills are performed on each aseptic filling line twice a year. Additional tests can be performed to evaluate changes in procedures, practices, cleanroom equipment configurations, changes in HVAC conditions, installation of new HEPA filters, etc.

A question commonly asked is what is the magic of three batches in a validation program. The number three is used because it could be said that one is equal to an event, two equals coincidence and three is equal to science. Three is a rough optimum for capturing variability at an acceptable cost. Therefore, the magic number three is a reasonable approach to demonstrate reproducibility of any line.

During the fill, the quality department should be the primary observing group. In addition, videotaping has become widely accepted as a method of review (in the case of any failures) and training.

All personnel must be gown plated on exit. At a minimum, gloves and forearms must be tested. Any positive results must be identified and investigated.

Interpretation of Results and Acceptance Criteria

Despite the number of units filled during a process simulation test, or the number of positives allowed, the ultimate goal for the number of positives in any process simulation is zero! A sterile product is, after all, one that contains no viable organisms.

The following criteria should be used to establish appropriate process simulation test limits and acceptance criteria:

■ The test methodology must simulate the process as closely as possible. Deviations from the established processes must be justified.

■ The rationale for choosing the methodology and limits must be justified and documented.

■ Test methodology should be sensitive enough to confirm a low process simulation test contamination rate and the selection limit must be routinely achievable.

■ Any positive unit indicates a potential problem regardless of run size. All positives should be identified and should result in a thorough and documented investigation.

In the "Guidance for Industry FDA Sterile Drug Products Produced by Aseptic Processing" on 30 September 2004 the following interpretation of test results is indicated.

■ One filling fewer than 5000 units: no contamination should be detected.

■ One filling from 5000 to 10,000 units: one contaminate in a unit should result in an investigation, including consideration of a repeat media fill. Two contaminated units are considered cause for revalidation following investigation.

■ When filling more than 10,000 units: one contaminated unit should result in an investigation. Two contaminated units are considered cause for revalidation following investigation.

■ For any size, intermittent incidents of microbial contamination in media filled lines can be indicative of a persistent low-level contamination problem that should be investigated. Accordingly, reoccurring incidents of contaminated units in media fills for an individual line, regardless of acceptance criteria, would be a signal of an adverse trend on the aseptic processing line that should lead to problem identification, correction, and revalidation.

Failure Investigation and Corrective Action

A contaminated container should be carefully examined for any breach in the integrity of the container system. Damaged containers should not be considered an evaluation (acceptance) of an aseptic processing capability of the process. However, a vial that is broken during incubation should be addressed.

All positives from integral containers should be identified to at least genus and species whenever possible. A comprehensive consistent sampling and identification scheme is crucial in the investigation and determination of the contamination source. This is the same practice that is performed for all ISO 5 and sterility testing suites.

Identify the contaminant and compare the result to the database of the organisms most recently identified. Processing records should be reviewed. Critical systems should be reviewed and documented for changes. Calibration records should be checked. All HEPA filters in the filling area should be inspected and decertified if warranted. Personnel involved in the fill should be assessed to assure the proper training was provided. Validation and change control records should be reviewed for any procedure or process changes.

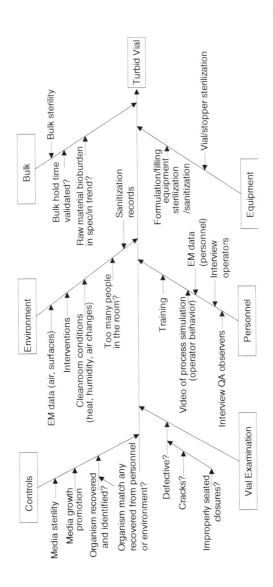

FIGURE 1 A fishbone analysis showing undesired event and the underlying fault events. *Abbreviation:* EM, environment monitoring.

A full risk analysis should be performed. A media failure signals an underlying weakness of the system or the process. In the context of GMP, a risk analysis focuses on what a failure means to the patient and, secondarily, to the particular manufacturing process and elements within the quality system.

The risk of contamination to an aseptic process by airborne contaminants entered through the air handling system to the facility is minimal. This is made evident by the fact that the data generated by the environmental monitoring program generally show zero microbial contaminants in an ISO Class 5 cleanroom or better and very low particulate (nonviable) contaminants. Any excursion should be investigated and documented; however, a variance is not an automatic invalidation of a process simulation test.

The major source, however, of contamination in the cleanroom is widely accepted to be the personnel that are present. Use of a cleanroom does not guarantee sterility nor prevent contamination caused by poor operator aseptic techniques, poor gowning practices, and lack of training. This contamination, however, is nonrandom in nature and must be strongly correlated with human activity.

A fishbone analysis shows an undesired event and then determines the underlying fault events that could contribute to it (Fig. 1). The final investigation report should contain the following:

- A summary of the occurrence
- All systems investigated, not just the systems tied to the failure
- A conclusion as to the cause and supporting documentation
- Potential effect on previous batches since last media fill
- Corrective action
- Outcome of additional process simulation tests if they were performed
- Appropriate signatures

This investigation needs to be completed in a timely fashion. It may be necessary to issue an interim report (9).

Three consecutive successful process simulations are required to qualify a new or significantly revised change aseptic line or area. If there has been a failure on any process simulation without an assignable cause, one process simulation is required for requalification of an aseptic processing line.

Invalidation of a Media Fill

A media fill can only be invalidated for reasons that would absolutely result in the discard of a product batch. These conditions must be filled out explicitly and the written justification for the media fill discard and the decision should be made on the day of execution.

Under what conditions may a process simulation be invalidated?

- Failure of growth promotion of media, provided there are no positive units in the process simulation.
- Failure of physical conditions in the aseptic processing area (power outage, pressurization loss, HEPA filter failure).
- Failure of operators to follow proper procedures not permitted in normal production which would lead to the discontinuation of a batch and rejection of all vials filled to that point.

Process simulation can be aborted for any reason when according to the procedure would lead to the discontinuation of a production batch. However, clear documentation of the event that caused the discontinuation should be performed and maintained. Process simulations can be invalidated for any or all of the above reasons.

CASE STUDY

In a paper presented by John Lindsey at the 2004 PDA Sitek Summit 8–20 March 2004, Orlando, Florida entitled "Media Fill Challenges," case studies were presented of work that was done during the PDA aseptic processing course. The case studies indicated that the line had been contaminated and yet the media fill results in some cases had passed.

During Dr. Lindsey's case studies, filling line, the cleanroom, filling equipment, stoppable, sterile alcohol, and crimper, among others, were contaminated. The results of this study showed that in many of the cases, the media fills have passed, even though items had been severely compromised.

Five conclusions established at the summit that need to be considered are the following:

1. The level of environmental contamination can influence the sterility assurance of the product.
2. Good aseptic technique can reduce the risk to the product contamination even in the presence of a contaminated environment.
3. Personnel are the main vectors of contamination in an aseptically filling facility, unless a contaminated aerosol is created.
4. A contaminated media fill unit is a major event in modern cleanrooms with basic design, including HEPA filtered air, and a knowledge of good aseptic techniques of positive filled media vial or product filled vial should never occur.
5. Any positive filled unit, regardless of the number of vials, should be investigated thoroughly and if a reasonable, assignable cause is not determined, the results should be considered a failure.

SUMMARY

The primary purpose for a media fill program is to demonstrate the capability of the aseptic process to produce a sterile product. The regulatory requirements, the detailed planning and execution, and the careful documentation are all designed to support this single goal.

Media fills will also provide an important opportunity to train, certify, and maintain certification of employees working in product manufacture. This in turn supports the sterility assurance of the product but is an important enough secondary goal to stand alone.

Training of employees supports not only the specific process being simulated but also the enhancement of the individual's aseptic technique skills overall. Together these two goals are mandated by the regulatory authorities to comply with current good manufacturing practices.

FDA has focused attention on media fill programs as part of a risk based approach that places more scrutiny in areas of higher risk to the patient population. FDA requires that media fill simulations be designed to represent the actual manufacturing practices and process, and concentrate on factors that are most likely to result in failure, including "worst-case scenarios."

CONCLUSIONS

- Media fills are a necessary part of validation of aseptic processing and ongoing routine monitoring.
- Microbial contamination of sterile products manufactured by aseptic processing is mainly caused by human interventions.
- Regardless of the number of positives recovered from a media fill, it is the duty of manufacturers to investigate the origin of microbial contamination to ensure that both the aseptic manufacturing environment and the product are not at risk.

Media fills in practical numbers have the capability only of detecting contamination which is related to events which may compromise asepsis and not of estimating the underlying contamination rate of the process operating under stochastic control (10).

FURTHER READING

ISO 13408-1. Aseptic Processing of health care products-Part 1: General Requirements, First Edition, 1998-08-01.
PDA. Current practices in the validation of aseptic processing. Technical Report Number 36, 2001.

REFERENCES

1. FDA. Current good manufacturing practices for finished pharmaceuticals. Federal Register 43, 29 September 1978:45077.
2. Code of Federal Regulations 21 CFR Part 211.113(b).
3. FDA. Guideline on sterile drug products produced by aseptic processing, 1987.
4. Roganti F, Boeh RJ. Design of an aseptic process simulation. Pharm Technol September 2004, Page 76–84.
5. Parenteral Drug Association. Validation of a septic filling for solution drug products. Technical Monograph Number 2, Philadelphia, Pennsylvania, 1980.
6. High purity water systems.
7. Agalloco J. Managing aseptic interventions. Pharm Technol March 2005, page 56–66.
8. Kawamura K, Abe H. A novel approach to the statistical evaluation of media fill tests by the difference from no contamination data. PDA Journal, Vol 58, No. 6, November-December 2004:309–320.
9. PDA Technical Report Number 22. Process simulation testing for aseptically filled products, 1996 Supplement; 50(S1).
10. Halls NA. Practicalities of setting acceptance criteria for media fill trials. PDA J 2000 May–June ; Lyon 54(3):247–251.

7 Water Monitoring

Anne Marie Dixon and Karen Zink McCullough

7 Water Monitoring

Anne Marie Dixon
Cleanroom Management Associates, Inc., Carson City, Nevada, U.S.A.

Karen Zink McCullough
Whitehouse Station, New Jersey, U.S.A.

INTRODUCTION

Water is ubiquitous in the pharmaceutical industry. It is used as a support component [clean in place (CIP), presterilization preparation of vials and stoppers] as well as a major raw material in formulations. Microorganisms may be isolated from the purification, storage, and distribution portions of any water system. If water is used in the final product, these microorganisms or their byproducts may create a significant patient risk. Control of a water system is established through careful validation and the setting of specifications [temperature, total organic carbon (TOC), conductivity, flow rater, microbial load, endotoxin] that govern the routine operation of the system. Once validated, control of the system is demonstrated by careful and regular monitoring of the physical parameters of the system (volume, temperature, etc.) as well as the quality attributes of the water that is produced.

STANDARDS

Water quality specifications for a number of types of water used in the pharmaceutical industry are defined by the U.S. Pharmacopeia (USP) and other international organizations. The standards listed in the "Official Monographs/Water" of the USP are enforceable by the U.S. Food and Drug Administration (FDA). The FDA defines good manufacturing practices for the healthcare industry (pharmaceuticals, biologicals, and medical device) for the production and use of pharmaceutical waters including regulation of the facilities that house water production systems. FDA has published a document entitled "Guide to Inspections of High-Purity Water Systems." This document, while intended to be used as a guide for FDA investigators, provides information for industry on the agency's expectations for the design and operation of systems that produce pharmaceutical grade water.

To meet regulatory concerns is to demonstrate control over the process. This is accomplished by proper specifications for design, validation, operation, and monitoring. In addition, testing procedures, operating and maintenance protocols and procedures, and accurate record keeping are all important components of the overall process established to consistently produce quality compendial water.

VALIDATION

Validation will ensure that the systems meet the required quality standards. Validation of a water system includes the installation qualification (IQ), operational qualification (OQ), and performance qualification (PQ).

The purpose of the IQ is to identify each piece of equipment in or component of the system to determine that the installation is as per approved specifications. The IQ must demonstrate the following:

- The system was designed and built according to specifications.
- The equipment performance is within specifications and is the system that was tested by the manufacturer.
- All components are properly installed and the utilities are consistent with the equipment requirements.
- The operators have been properly trained in the correct operation of the equipment.
- The equipment and monitoring instrumentation are as per the specifications.
- The system is housed under the proper environmental conditions.

The IQ documentation package should include a description of the system and full detailed drawings. The process and instrumentation diagram (P&ID) is a key document. It must be a clear, concise, and accurate reflection of the as-built condition. The P&ID is used during the IQ to check the equipment installation and "walk down" the pipe routing. The P&ID is also the source of sample port numbering and locations that are tested throughout the PQ and beyond.

After the equipment and piping have been verified, installed, and operational, the initial phase of testing can begin, generally in the OQ portion of the validation. The objective of the OQ is to ensure that the tested system performances are consistent with the process for which it was intended. Therefore, during the OQ, the equipment, cycles, and programs must be tested to prove that the system functions according to specifications.

Initial sanitization is critical, as is the continued sanitization of a loop. If the loop is kept hot, routine sanitization can follow standard practice but ambient loops or drops downstream of a heat exchanger can be a challenge. Challenges to maintaining water systems at points of use include the ability to sanitize the sampling ports, ease of sample taking, proximity to a drain for adequate flush, and dead legs.

FDA is very concerned that the microbiological and chemical samples are taken in the same manner (e.g., through hoses) as the system is used. So, there needs to be considerable control over the sterilization and changing of hoses along with procedural constraints on their use (e.g., draining, not touching the floor, etc.). All users of the water system including manufacturing operators and water samplers must be trained on the same standard operating procedure (SOP) for water procurement to assure that procurement practices are consistent and appropriate to the intended use of the water produced by the system.

The PQ is designed to demonstrate that the water system will consistently produce quality water over an extended period of time—usually no less than one year. During the course of that year, any seasonal variations in the quality of the feed water and operating parameters could affect the quality of the water. For example, in the spring, especially in the northeast portion of the United States, increases in Gram-negative organisms have been observed. Any water system must be designed to operate under anticipated extremes. Therefore, the "whole" system from pretreatment to deionization to distillation to distribution must perform to specifications in production conditions at all times. The final part of the validation is the compilation of the data into a final report.

During the initial month or 90 days of the PQ, samples are taken daily from all points on the loop and are tested for quality attributes (TOC, conductivity, endotoxin, microbial load). As experience is gained with the system and confidence in the system's ability to consistently produce quality water is built, sampling may be reduced incrementally, but must be representative of all segments of the system. Ultimately, a routine monitoring plan will emerge from the analysis of PQ data. Minimally, routine monitoring should assure that each loop and the holding tanks are sampled once a day and that each port on the loop is sampled at least once a week. The reduction in sampling is justified if the PQ data have demonstrated stability in the quality of the water in the loop and have also demonstrated that each of the ports consistently operated properly (i.e., no leaks, no mechanical problems with valves, no dead legs, sufficient flushing). Once the "hardware" of the system (piping and ports) have been qualified as operating properly and consistently, one might assume that water sampled from any port on the recirculation loop is representative of the quality of the water in the loop. The requirement to do each port once a week is to monitor the port, especially if there are changes to the configuration or tubing or something else external to the actual quality of the water post-still.

SAMPLING

Once in operation, control is monitored by the periodic taking of samples and testing the samples against the specifications set during validation. Monitoring actually serves three purposes:

1. In the absence of excursions, data gathered from monitoring demonstrate stability of the system.
2. Sudden increases in one or more of the system specifications (e.g., increase in endotoxin or microbial load) may be indicative of an acute problem such as failure of reverse osmosis (RO) membranes.
3. Long-term gradual increases in detected levels or numbers of excursions in one or more of the system specifications could signal a chronic problem such as the establishment of a biofilm.

The key to any qualification or monitoring activity is the integrity of the samples. In-line testing by calibrated instrumentation eliminates the need for "grab" samples and provides assurance that sample integrity is maintained and data are accurate. However, when analysts have to take samples, and when sampling sometimes occurs in uncontrolled or nonsterile support areas for aseptic processing, sample integrity is easily breached. Therefore, a few simple but very important precautions are required.

Sample Vessel

Sample vessels must be prepared in a manner that suits their use:

■ Samples taken for microbial limits (bioburden) analysis must be sterile. If containers are prepared in-house, their sterilization either in the autoclave or in a dry heat oven must be validated.
■ Vessels used for specimens undergoing endotoxin analysis must be free of interferences such as detectable endotoxin and inhibitory leachables. If these containers are prepared in-house they must be subject to a validated dry heat

depyrogenation cycle (autoclaving is not a method for the depyrogenation of glass or plastic containers.) If vessels are purchased as disposable, sterile, and "pyrogen-free," USP < 85 > requires that they be prescreened for the presence of interferences—residual endotoxin on surfaces and/or inhibitory substances that could be leached from plastics (1). Plastics are suitable for sampling if they have been shown to be noninterfering with the test. As a general rule, polypropylene should not be used to draw samples for endotoxin testing as inhibitors from the plastic surface have been detected and reported in the literature (2,3). If a certificate of analysis is accepted for residual endotoxin or inhibitory substances in sample containers, it must be verified as acceptable either by "in-house" confirmation or by a directed vendor audit.

■ Containers used for obtaining samples for TOC analysis must be scrupulously cleaned of organic residues and must have a tight fitting lid.

Samples for microbial limits, endotoxin, or TOC testing are easily contaminated and must be taken very carefully to avoid extrinsic contamination. In a nonsterile area or uncontrolled area, the sampler must take care not to touch the inside of the container or lid and must not expose the inside of the lid or container to dirty surfaces (e.g., do not lay the lid down on a dirty surface, do not touch the end of the drop to the inside of the container or the lid). Water must be allowed to flow freely, and it is collected from the stream, being careful not to touch the inside of the container to the outside of the sampling port. Care must be taken to avoid using alcohol to clean the end of a drop prior to taking a TOC sample, as residual disinfectant could contaminate the sample.

FDA's "Guide to the Inspection of High-Purity Water Systems" requires that at any point of use sampling reflect how the water is to be drawn during manufacture (4). For example, if water for manufacturing is routinely drawn through sterile tubing, the monitoring sample must be drawn through the very same tubing. Care must be taken by both manufacturing and sampling personnel to reduce the possibility of contamination from tubing by:

■ Letting the tubing drain freely when not in use so as not to provide "puddles" of standing water inside of the tubing for microorganisms to grow.
■ Keeping the outlet end of the tubing from touching the floor or hands.

If contamination of the tubing during manufacturing or sampling is suspected, the tubing should be discarded and a new piece of sterile tubing should be installed. Tubing should be changed regularly depending on the quality attributes and intended use of the product. Clearly, sterility and asepsis are more important for parenterals than for nonsterile active pharmaceutical ingredients (APIs).

It is important to design the system in a manner that provides for unobstructed access to all sampling ports. Ports that are behind or under formulation vessels, in closets, or are situated 9 ft above the ground are difficult to sample, and their placement only increases the risk of contamination upon sampling their placement may but also pose a significant safety risk to the operator.

Prior to taking the sample, a volume of water is flushed to waste. The total volume of this flush or the total time of the flush must be validated. The purpose of the flush is to eliminate any potential contaminants from the inside of the sample port. The flush is an important step in any sample taking, but is especially important in an ambient system where any length of a deadleg is a potential site for the seeding of a biofilm.

Sample volume for microbiological analysis should be reflective of the expected quality of the water and the type of analysis to be performed. Water for injection has a microbial limit of 10 CFU/100 mL. Because of the expected low numbers, a sample size of less than 100 mL is unacceptable for water for injection (WFI) or for any sterile water. Potable water used as feed for further purification or nonsterile purified water used in the formulation of nonparenteral preparations will have microorganisms, so a sample size of 10, 1, or even 1 mL of a 1:10 dilution of the sample may be appropriate depending on the expected microbial load. The real concern for WFI is endotoxin. WFI can pass the limulus amebocyte lysate (LAL) endotoxin test yet fail microbial limits; conversely, WFI can fail the LAL endotoxin test yet pass microbial limits. It is therefore important to monitor the WFI system for both endotoxin in microorganisms.

Once the sample is taken, it must be transported back to the analysis laboratory in a method that will not compromise its integrity. Samples for TOC must have little or no headspace, samples for endotoxin and microbial limits must have caps firmly screwed on or snapped on. Once in the laboratory, analysis should commence as quickly as possible—usually within four hours of drawing the sample. Maximum time and optimum temperature for storage of samples not tested immediately must be validated, but samples for microbial limits and endotoxin should be refrigerated to slow any microbial growth. Freezing of samples for microbial limits testing or endotoxin testing is not advised unless validated.

ROUTINE MONITORING

A pharmaceutical system is dynamic and thus requires ongoing microbiological monitoring. After the initial validation, the three elements of a microbiological monitoring program for a water system are:

1. Representative sampling
2. Investigative testing
3. Analyzing the resulting data

Trending is an effective way to analyze data from a dynamic water system. The results of the trend analysis become the driving force for determining the best approach to ongoing sample testing. For example, seasonal differences in feed water might be reflected in an upward trend for microbial counts the pretreatment system. This increasing trend will likely have two immediate effects: (i) it precipitates discussion on increasing the frequency maintenance and regeneration of the pretreatment system during certain times of the year and (ii) it will provide a focus for the investigation of a distillation or distribution failure. Monitoring accomplished by trend analysis can provide a continuous quality improvement process for water system control.

The microbiological quality attributes of a water system are measured by quantitative (total microbial and endotoxin) and qualitative methods (species identification, and presence or absence of coliform). The data must be reviewed in respect to the validation process specifications.

From a microbiological standpoint, any count is a potentially significant count. Given that bacteria would rather grow on a substrate than be suspended, the total number of bacteria that inhabit a system, particularly an ambient system, can be grossly underestimated by counting only planktonic (suspended) bacteria. Additionally, the testing technique can also underestimate the number of bacteria that truly inhabit the system. Today, high-purity water is generally tested using low nutrient media to mimic the conditions under which these organisms grow. The detection of gram-negative bacteria in the system could be a foreshadowing of endotoxin problems.

All microbiological test methods must be validated. Data comparability over time will largely depend on the stability and robustness of the test method. As changes to the method may introduce additional variability in the test data, any modification should be thoughtfully considered and carefully validated.

Classical microbial monitoring, however, does not provide for real-time data. Depending on the test method and medium used, incubation times will extend up to five days. The bacterial endotoxins test provides accurate data in an hour or less that can be used as a monitoring tool or can be used as a "go/no go" decision on a tank full of formulation water. Rapid methods for the enumeration of live bacteria are currently available. These tests provide useable data, generally within four hours of taking the sample. Though not yet utilized as in-line monitoring systems, the use of these rapid methods is a giant step in the application of technology to the concept of continuous monitoring or process analytical technology (PAT).

To develop an effective microbiological monitoring plan, the intended purpose must be defined. The monitoring program must allow for the demon-stration of:

- The quality of the water as used
- The evaluation of the system stability over time (ongoing system evaluation through trend analysis)
- Compliance

The quality plan for the water system must provide for the development of sampling and testing protocols that will provide data to support the monitoring plan. The continuous evaluation and re-evaluation of the number of different sites to sample and of the frequency of sampling at each site are dependent on the results of the trending.

Careful data organization and analysis including an assessment both of the severity of each individual excursion and its possible association with a develop-ing system or trend will help to identify an appropriate and effective corrective action in the event of a microbiological excursion. The sampling plan must be flexible and dynamic enough to respond to evolving patterns and trends. The following conditions might influence the sampling plan:

- Change in sanitization methodology or frequency
- Changes in sanitization effectiveness
- Regeneration frequency of deionization beds
- Effectiveness of microbial retentive filters
- Detection of still leakage or malfunction
- Detection of equipment failures

INVESTIGATIONS

The failure of a water system to meet any specification is a serious business and compliance concern. Failures in the system during the PQ of the system are of particular concern because any anomalies in the design or functioning of the sys-tem should have been detected and corrected in the execution of the design qualification (DQ), IQ, and OQ of the system. By the time PQ is executed, the system, whether generating purified water, water for injection, or of a site-specific water quality, should be working optimally.

Failure modes based on quality attributes and specifications for the water generated by pharmaceutical systems include chemical problems (TOC, conductivity), biological problems (microbial load, endotoxin), or nonviable particulates. Inability to validate and maintain the efficient cleaning of the system can lead to increased levels of any of these attributes.

Each excursion must be investigated to determine the root cause. Arguably, a failure during qualification is more critical than a routine failure, as this is the time when the system has to "prove" its ability to produce water of consistently high quality.

Because of the importance of any failure, and particularly the importance of repeated failures or patterns of excursions, a thorough investigation is warranted. Sometimes, even the most robust investigation will not reveal any obvious root cause. However, even though a root cause might be difficult to identify, it does not relieve a firm of the responsibility of performing an unbiased, scientific, and timely investigation into any water system failure.

At a very high level, the investigation must start with the identification of all of the possible failure routes or modes that could have contributed to the excursion. Even if a member of the investigation team feels strongly that he or she can identify the root cause without an investigation, it is important that all possibilities be either eliminated or elevated by performing an objective analysis.

A tool such as a fishbone diagram makes the start of the investigation easy and allows the investigation team to systematically work through the problem. A good place to start the investigation is to map out the system using the "as-built" drawings and walk through the component parts to identify all of the critical control points where the failure could have been introduced. At the "head" of the fish is the description of the failure (e.g., endotoxin, TOC, conductivity, microbial limit). The "bones" of the fish identify all of the possible routes to that failure. In this case,

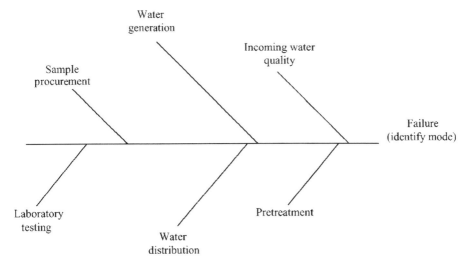

FIGURE 1 Fishbone diagram of investigation.

incoming water quality, pretreatment, water generation, water distribution, water procurement, and water testing have all been identified as possible causes of the failure (Fig. 1).

INCOMING WATER

The quality of the incoming water is critical to the choice of treatment processes and controls required to create consistently high-quality water for manufacturing purposes. Water quality can be seasonal, with higher microbial counts and higher endotoxin often showing up in warmer weather. Testing of incoming water is an important part of the control of a water system, but an understanding of the water source and any treatment of the water at the source are also important. For example, a firm will want to get certificates of analysis for the water from a municipal water provider so that (i) there is an understanding of what happens to the water between the source and the plant and (ii) there is an understanding of what

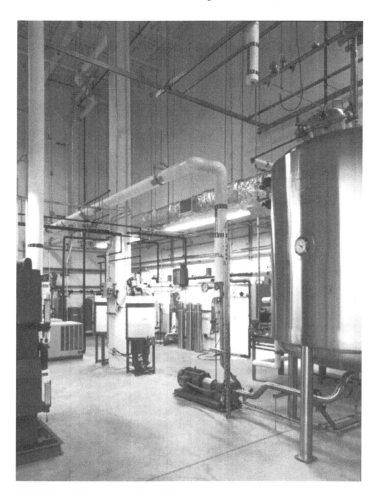

FIGURE 2 Water plant with holding tank.

needs to be incorporated into the in-house treatment system to mitigate fluctuations in municipal water quality.

PRETREATMENT

The pretreatment is a very important but often overlooked part of the water system. Mathematical models of water systems indicate that the quality of the incoming water, the efficiency of each of the pretreatment steps, and the frequency of cleaning/regeneration of mixed media and charcoal as well as deionized (water) (DI) beds are vital to the production of consistently good quality water.

■ Look at the quality of the incoming potable water—has it changed over time? City water does change—is your problem associated with a change?

■ Look for loading in pretreatment filtration systems including charcoal filters and deionization beds. Microorganisms can set up house in these systems and produce not only more organisms, but also in the case of Gram-negative organisms, colonized pretreatment components can be endotoxin factories.

■ Look at maintenance records for charcoal filters and deionization beds—were regeneration events missed? Have regeneration methods been validated? Has the regeneration interval been validated? Are regeneration events spaced too far apart?

■ If a UV light is part of pretreatment, is it functioning properly? Testing pre- and post-UV exposure should be done as part of the qualification of the system and at specified intervals.

■ If RO is part of the pretreatment process, it must be validated for its intended use.

WATER GENERATION

Given the mechanism of distillation, a properly functioning still should consistently generate WFI—i.e., water that is sterile and has an endotoxin content under 0.25 EU/mL. Still efficiency must be validated during OQ and monitored closely for a year during PQ. Care must be taken during normal operation that the efficiency of the still is not exceeded due to poor pretreatment. Failures post still should initiate investigation on validation of the still as well as the quality of the water upstream to study the possibility of still overloading.

If water for manufacturing is generated using only RO rather than by distillation, particular care must be taken to examine the process flow for the following:

■ RO membranes must be in series, to provide a "safety net" in the case that one membrane is damaged or exhibits microbial grow through.

■ As with the still, the efficiency of the RO membrane series and the system's preventive maintenance requirements including sanitization and/or membrane replacement intervals must be identified and validated during qualification.

WATER DISTRIBUTION

The distribution system, consisting of the holding tank for the generated water, the piping, and the sample/use ports, is perhaps the must vulnerable in the entire generation/distribution/use cycle.

In general, to keep the possibility of bacterial contamination and growth at a minimum, distribution systems must be engineered to keep the water circulating. Dead legs, which provide an environment for the accumulation of noncirculating

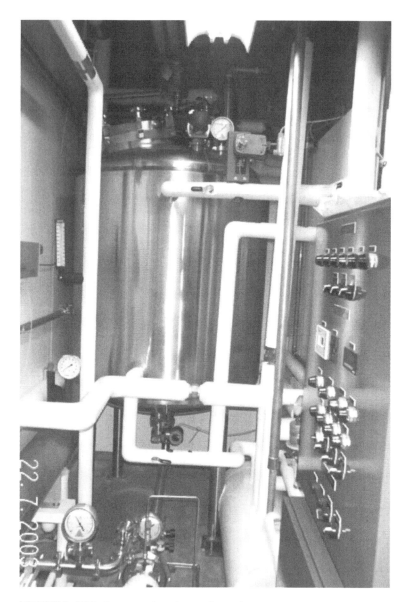

FIGURE 3 WFI storage tank and control panels.

water and the growth of bacteria, are to be avoided. Sample and use ports must be
accessible and sanitary. Piping must be constructed free of rough welds, which can
act as a home for bacteria and a starting point for rouging in the system. Sampling
valves including gaskets must be made of inert materials that are resistant to corrosion
and degradation by the constant exposure to deionized water and/or the port sanitization method. Physical conditions that provide a place for bacterial growth are
unacceptable in any type of purified water system.

The system's holding tank for water immediately downstream of the still is a place where contamination will lead to the fouling of the entire system. Maintenance of the tank in a sanitized state is essential. Proper venting and the use of sterile vent filters on the tank will greatly reduce the possibility of the introduction of bacteria into the headspace of the tank when water is drawn for distribution. If air or an inert gas is used as an overlay for the tank water, its must be validated such that it will not contribute either viable or nonviable particulates to the water; essentially, the overlay must meet the classification of the area into which it is introduced or the substance for which it is used as an overlay (Aseptic Processing Guideline, 2004). Because water in a circulating system is returned to the tank, an understanding of the quality of the water returned and the effect of its reintroduction on the overall quality of the water already in the tank must be understood during the qualification phase of the system.

Because of the nature of bacteria to grow on solid substrates, biofilms are of particular concern in cold or ambient systems as well as downstream of any heat exchanger unit on a hot system. Sanitization of the system, whether hot or cold, must be validated. Sanitizing agent(s), time and temperature of exposure and the sanitization interval of the piping, sampling ports, use ports, and the holding tank are all enormously important to maintaining the quality of a pharmaceutical water system. Any lack of validation, lack of preventive maintenance that will keep the system in a validated state, or departure from the validated conditions is likely to be a root cause for a water failure.

Some ambient systems are particularly vulnerable to microbial contamination, RO or other filtration methods that operate at ambient temperature and are susceptible to contamination and microbial growth, which compromises the entire downstream distribution system.

SAMPLE PROCUREMENT

Water procurement procedures, particularly the analyst's water sampling technique and equipment used to take a failed sample, are almost always the first of many areas called into question. While this is understandable because it is the "easiest" to explain, it is important to recognize that the laboratory is only one of many root causes and should be one of many paths that are studied during the course of the investigation.

If documented evidence can be produced that implicates either the sampler or the equipment, then the sample result may be legitimately voided, corrective/preventive action identified, and a new sample taken. Examples of these kinds of acute errors are an acknowledgement by the sampler that the sample could have been compromised due to lack of aseptic technique, leaving the sampling vessels open for more time than necessary, not flushing the port for the validated amount of time, and inappropriate sterilization/depyrogenation of the sampling vessels. If trend analysis suggests a more chronic problem, e.g., a lot of purchased vessels that are nonsterile, a majority of the excursions assigned to one sampler, an unvalidated test method, or a sampling vessel whose chemical properties inhibit the proper testing of the sample, then the action taken become more preventive than corrective:

- Examine the training courses and records of the analysts involved.
- If a single sampler seems to have more excursions than others, go out and observe the analyst's technique.

- Go out and walk the system—are the ports in question particularly difficult to access? Does port configuration require that the sampler sacrifice aseptic technique for safety? Are the ports dripping or do they appear to be compromised?
- Examine sampling materials—is there a particular lot or manufacturer of sampling vessel that is implicated?

The implications of "false"positive due to a sampling error is huge, as the integrity of the system is in doubt unless and until a sampling or testing error can be conclusively identified.

SAMPLE TESTING

A firm needs to assure itself that the integrity of a sample is not compromised between the time it is taken and the time it is tested. In terms of the chain of custody of the sample:

- How was the sample transported?
- Who transported it? Is this a different person than the analyst who drew the sample?
- Where and under what conditions was the sample stored prior to testing?
- Have those storage conditions been validated?
- Could the integrity of the sample have been compromised by something physical (e.g., loose top on the sampling vessel, labeling mix ups)?

The laboratory investigation must proceed past the procurement and transport/storage issues and look carefully at the practices of the laboratory and the laboratory analysts:

- Is the test method validated?
- Did the procedure used in failed test depart from the validated test method?
- Was the analyst properly trained and qualified?
- Was the test equipment appropriately prepared (e.g., sterile materials for bioburden testing, depyrogenated materials for endotoxin testing, and clean vessels for TOC and nonviable particulates)?
- If the testing was performed under a controlled environmental condition, is there evidence that the environment met the requirements necessary for testing?

All of the items of the failure investigation as defined above, when identified and reviewed, will lead to a completed study with an accurate root cause and corrective actions or preventive actions, or both.

As stated at the beginning of this chapter, water is a critical utility. Attention must be paid to every detail in the design, installation, operations, and preventative maintenance of a system.

FURTHER READING

FDA Guide to Inspections of High-Purity Water Systems.
United States Pharmacopeia 29⟨1231⟩. "Water for Pharmaceutical Purposes". The United States Pharmacopeial Convention, Rockville, Maryland, 2006.
U.S. EPA 40CFR141.21 Total Coliform Rule.

REFERENCES

1. United States Pharmacopeia 29(85), "Bacterial Endotoxin Test". The United States Pharmacopeial Convention, Rockville, Maryland, 2006.
2. Associates of Cape Cod. The problems with plastics. LAL Update 1988; 6(3):1–3.
3. Roslansky PF, Dawson ME, Novitsky TJ. Plastics, endotoxins, and the limulus amebocyte lysate test. J Parent Sci Technol 1991; 45(2):83–87.
4. Food and Drug Administration. Guide to inspections of high purity water systems, 1993. http://www.fda.gov/ora/inspect ref/igs/high.html.

8 Bacterial Endotoxin Testing

Karen Zink McCullough

Bacterial Endotoxin Testing

Karen Zink McCullough

Whitehouse Station, New Jersey, U.S.A.

INTRODUCTION

Why is a chapter on the bacterial endotoxin test (BET) included in a book on environmental monitoring? Because endotoxins, which are potent pyrogens, or fever causing agents, are by-products of viable and/or nonviable contamination of parenteral products by Gram-negative microorganisms. If we define a drug product's "environment" as the combination of raw materials or active pharmaceutical ingredients (APIs) and their related processing environments, drug product manufacturing steps and their related environments, and laboratory testing and its related environment, we can demonstrate that major sources of Gram-negative contamination in the parenteral industry are environmental and include but may not be limited to the following:

- Acute and chronic problems with water systems and distribution loops
- Raw materials and APIs, especially those obtained from natural sources
- Nonvalidated cleaning and/or storage of manufacturing equipment
- Nonvalidated hold times for nonsterile product formulations
- Nonvalidated depyrogenation procedures
- By-products of fermentations
- Shedding of microorganisms by operators, and
- The technique, equipment, and reagents used in the performance of the test itself

The control of endotoxin in parenterals is not accomplished through end-product testing, but is assured through careful system and process validation, value-added process control and thorough operator training. A validated test system and properly qualified analysts and an understanding of the benefits and limitations of the test method are essential to an accurate test result.

> There was no evaluation or report of evaluation of the process from a pyrogen/endotoxin aspect. —FDA 483 citation

The risks of not monitoring a drug product's environment to both patient welfare and a firm's "bottom line" are clear. As with the sterility test, a final endotoxin determination based solely on a retrospective analysis of a statistically insignificant number of units at the end-product testing stage could result in the release of product that is contaminated. The risk to the patient is a potentially severe febrile reaction or even death. The risk to the firm is a recall and possible legal and compliance actions. Conversely, a "false positive" result on a finished product test due to nonvalidated or improperly validated test methods, uncontrolled test conditions, or unqualified analysts could cause firm to reject a batch of product that is well within specification and would pose no risk to the patient.

Carefully conceived validation and process control rooted in a risk-based model makes sense in the following:

- Reducing the risk of hazards to the patient
- Reducing the risk of product liability
- Reducing the risk of compliance actions against the drug product manufacturer
- Reducing the risk of potentially unnecessary financial losses to the firm due to false positive results
- Reducing time and money spent on non value-added validation studies
- Reducing the level of monitoring to a minimum but efficient and valuable level

In "Pharmaceutical current Good Manufacturing Practices (cGMPs) for the 21st Century," the Food and Drug Administration (FDA) has acknowledged that the increasing complexity in both the numbers and the types of parenteral products being manufactured and the globalization of the pharmaceutical industry have made the concept of "one size fits all" Good Manufacturing Practice (GMP) regulation inefficient and cumbersome (1,2). In that publication and subsequent updates, it is clear that the compliance focus is shifting away from a plethora of "GMP-isms" toward the concept of a Quality System, where firms take into account the intended use of the product, its specific formulation and processing steps, and its identified quality attributes. The implications of this initiative on the future of parenteral manufacturing are enormous. The days of blindly following a set of externally imposed rules and regulations will be replaced by a requirement to understand products and processes so that an internally determined and customized set of rules based on universally accepted best practices can be applied. FDA will require justification, articulation, implementation, and monitoring of these internal rules with an eye toward reassessment during the product life cycle and modification of testing and control as necessary.

This chapter will focus on the utilization of risk management in the application of cGMP/Quality System to the use of the BET as a tool for the proactive, detection, monitoring and control of endotoxins in drug-product manufacturing. For those readers who are new to endotoxin and endotoxin testing, the concepts presented in this chapter are based on the following facts and assumptions as described in the law (21 CFR), the science of endotoxin and its detection, and the compliance requirements for the utilization of the BET to detect endotoxin (3–6). Historical and technical explanations of these facts and assumptions may be found in the section "Peeling the Artichoke: Determination of critical control points (CCPs) in the Laboratory Performance of the BET Assay," as well as in a number of referenced texts.

1. The Law—GMPs and the Quality System Regulation (7–10):

- 21 CFR 211.167(a): "For each batch of drug product purporting to be sterile and/or pyrogen free, there shall be appropriate laboratory testing to determine conformance to such requirements."
- 21 CFR 211.100(a): "There shall be written procedures for production and process control designed to assure that the drug products have the identity, strength, quality and purity they purport or are represented to possess."
- 21 CFR 820.70(a): "Each manufacturer shall develop, conduct, control and monitor production processes to ensure that a device conforms to its specifications."

- 21 CFR 820.70(e): "Each manufacturer shall establish and maintain procedures to prevent contamination of equipment or product that could reasonably be expected to have an adverse effect on product quality."

2. The Science of pyrogen, endotoxin, and the BET (11,12):

- Pyrogens, by definition, are fever-causing substances.
- Endotoxins are a specific class of very potent pyrogens. Endotoxins are a structural component of the outer cell membrane of Gram-negative bacteria.
- If administered in sufficient quantities, patients can suffer a number of adverse effects from the intravenous injection of endotoxin. Excessive doses of endotoxin can be lethal.
- Endotoxin is a serious hazard in the pharmaceutical industry, as it is ubiquitous, is potent, and is difficult to remove.
- Endotoxin is not retained by sterilizing filters, nor is it consistently reduced or eliminated by moist heat (autoclaving) or irradiation (γ, e-beaming) sterilization methods (13,14).
- Endotoxin is remarkably heat-stable, requiring high heat for long periods of time for depyrogenation (13–15).
- Lipopolysaccharide is purified endotoxin.
- An endotoxin unit (EU) is a unit of measure of an endotoxin's biological activity, and not weight or mass.
- The BET is a highly specific and sensitive way to detect, monitor, and quantitate endotoxins in any raw material, in process sample or drug product.

3. Compendial and Compliance Definitions and Requirements (3–6):

- As of 2001, the JP, the EP, and the USP have published a "harmonized" BET. While some of the details of the test methods or language might differ among the three documents, they are philosophically aligned.
- An endotoxin limit is a calculation of the maximum level of endotoxin that can be safely administered in a dose of drug product without causing a fever in the patient. The endotoxin limit is based on the "threshold pyrogenic dose of endotoxin" determined experimentally in rabbits and confirmed in humans that is defined as 5 EU/kg (16,17). The formula for the endotoxin limit is K/M where K = the threshold pyrogenic limit of 5 EU/kg and M = dose/kg of patient weight/hr (18).
- Validation of the BET (also known as "inhibition/enhancement") is required for all materials under test (4–6,19,20). Test method validation of the BET requires the quantitative recovery of a known added amount of endotoxin (endotoxin "spike") to undiluted or diluted drug product, in process sample or raw material/excipient sample to demonstrate lack of test interference by the substance. Inhibition interference could result in a "false negative" test, and true enhancement interference (much more rare than inhibition) could result in a "false positive" test.

THE QUALITY SYSTEM

The Quality System, as defined in 21CFR 820, is the GMP regulation for the medical device industry (7). At the core of the Quality System is the recognition and clear articulation that control in manufacturing is a series of integrated and interdependent processes. The Quality System Regulation requires that each manufacturer establish and maintain a system of control over product and process that is appropriate for the quality attributes, product specifications and intended use of the final product.

The Quality System is comprised of seven essential and interdependent subsystems including management controls, facility and equipment controls, material controls, records/documents/change control controls, production and process controls including sterilization process controls, design controls, and corrective and preventive action (CAPA) (10,21). The purpose of the Quality System is to infuse quality, safety, and effectiveness into a product throughout its life cycle, starting with development and evolving as experience and data are gathered through routine manufacturing (22). At the core of the Quality System is the emphasis on solving quality problems through identification of CCPs, feedback, and analysis of data rather than a reliance on the pass/fail test results for finished product that dominate a traditional "quality control (QC)" model.

RISK

In "Pharmaceutical GMPs for the 21st Century," FDA has identified the concept of "risk management" as a convenient and appropriate tool for the application and implementation of the Quality System concept to parenteral manufacturing (1,2,23). The concept of risk is not a new one to FDA or other regulatory and industry trade organizations, but is new to the manufacture of small volume parenterals (SVPs) and large volume parenterals (LVPs) and biologics.

- 21CFR820: "Quality System Regulation" as applied to the manufacture of parenteral and nonparenteral medical devices requires a risk analysis as appropriate during device design validation [21 CFR 820.30 (g)].
- "Hazard Analysis and Critical Control Point Principles and Application Guidelines," published in 1997 by FDA, defines the principles of risk analysis as applied to processing in the food industry (24).
- "The European Parliament and the Council of the European Union" have published a directive on the manufacture of in vitro diagnostic (IVD) products (25). Annex 1 of this directive defines risk management as an essential requirement in the manufacture of IVD products.
- ISO 14971: "Medical Devices—Application of Risk Management to Medical Devices," describes a "framework within which experience, insight, and judgment are applied systematically to manage risks" (26).
- The European Diagnostic Manufacturers Association published a document entitled, "Risk Analysis of In vitro Diagnostic Medical Devices," which reminds readers that, "Acceptability cannot be generalized by means of a standard. Therefore, the manufacturer is obliged to consider the possible risks of the specific device during the development process in light of its intended use(s) and also taking account of potential manufacturer's liability" (27).

The basic tenet of risk management is that when one manages "risk" (the estimation of the possible occurrence of an identified hazard or hazardous condition), one understands, anticipates, and works to minimize the potential impact of a product failure, or hazard to the patient and to the manufacturer. A good risk-management program contains all of the components of a good Quality System from fundamental policies and task-specific procedures to change control to process validation and control to laboratory testing to release. For the process example in this chapter, the hazard is "endotoxin contamination," the failure mode is endotoxin in excess of the calculated or assigned endotoxin limit, and the implication of product failure to the patient is a potential severe adverse reaction (fever) or even death.

In order to understand, anticipate and minimize risk, one performs a "risk analysis" of product and process to identify critical steps in a process that, if uncontrolled, undetected, or incorrectly measured, could result in a product failure or patient hazard. Risk analysis, ideally, is based on a combination of empirical data, scientifically based assumptions, manufacturing experience, and compliance requirements. At the highest level in our example, once we calculate the endotoxin limit for the final product, we will be analyzing the drug-product environment for those places where endotoxin contamination might enter the system and where, by design, endotoxin is removed from the system. We define these steps or elements of the process as CCPs.

Ideally, risk analysis is undertaken by a cross-functional team of experts during the development phase of the drug-product life cycle, and is updated periodically to reflect any process improvements, formulation changes, equipment changes, etc. The risk team for endotoxin might consist of representatives from the following departments who understand the science and control of endotoxin: manufacturing, Quality Assurance (QA), engineering, maintenance, validation, QC microbiology (or QC chemistry if the BET is performed in an analytical laboratory), regulatory/compliance and development. Input from all team members will provide a comprehensive analysis of all aspects of the process including utilities, facilities, equipment, manufacturing steps, environment, and laboratory testing. Starting the analysis early in the product life cycle provides an opportunity to collect data for the exercise of setting appropriate limits for identified CCPs. However, risk analysis is also an extremely valuable exercise for the objective analysis of an existing process.

Setting limits for identified intermediate CCPs will provide the drug or device manufacturer with a significant measure of "risk control," in that the validation and routine monitoring schemes can be designed from the beginning to control endotoxin contamination and assure its removal where appropriate. Ultimately, the ability to assure the consistently high quality of the product is dependent on the firm's recognition of the importance of risk management, its commitment to periodically reassess risk, and its willingness make appropriate processing, control, and testing adjustments.

HAZARD AND CCP ANALYSIS

There are many published methods for risk analysis (22,24,26,28–30). While the choice of method and documentation is up to the user, comparison of all published methods for risk analysis indicates that even though approaches (example "top-down" vs. "bottom-up"), lexicons, charts, and diagrams may be different, they all rely on similar critical thinking processes (Table 1).

One method of applying the logic of risk management to parenteral manufacturing is through a method that FDA requires in the food industry called Hazard Analysis and Critical Control Point (HACCP) study (24). HACCP is a process-oriented approach to risk analysis, which focuses on prevention or reduction of risk through the proactive identification of critical points in the system (steps,

TABLE 1 Comparison of Three Different Methods of Risk Analysis

Objective	HACCP (22,24)	ISO 14971 (26)	FMEA (30)
Preparatory	Assemble a team, define a charter, and develop an HACCP Plan	Establish a risk management plan	Identifying FMEA elements
Define the problem relative to the intended use or purpose of the product and stated desirable or required quality characteristics	Principle 1: Conduct a hazard analysis	Risk analysis: Intended use/purpose; identification (ID) of quality characteristics; ID of known or forseeable hazards; estimation of risk for each hazard	Identify functions (intended purpose of the product); identify potential failure modes (categories of failure); define the effects or potential downstream consequences of failure mode
Establish critical priorities relative to the intended use or final specifications	Principle 2: Determine critical control points	Risk evaluation: Prioritization of risks	Quantify the severity of the effects; quantify the occurrence of the failure; calculate criticality (severity × occurrence)
Define limits for each critical step	Principle 3: Establish critical limits	Risk control: Option analysis; implementation of risk control measures	Define current design or process controls
Define monitoring parameters and consequences of excursion	Principle 4: Establish monitoring procedures	Risk control: Implementation of risk control measures	Determine and validate (if necessary) detection methods for monitoring
Validation, update as necessary according to change control	Principle 5: Establish corrective actions Principle 6: Establish verification procedures	Risk control: Verification of efficacy of the risk control measures. Overall residual risk evaluation, post production information	Reducing risk—revisit and provide feedback according to the controls and monitoring instituted
Documentation	Principle 7: establish record keeping	Risk management file	Document the study and actions taken

Abbreviations: HACCP, Hazard Analysis and Critical Control Point; ISO, International Standards Organization; FMEA, failure mode and effect analysis; ID, identification.

equipment, facilities, ingredients, methods, etc.), setting limits relative to the identified hazard, monitoring those limits, identifying possible CAPAs before an excursion happens, and documenting the entire program. There are seven basic principles to HACCP and they are as follows:

Principle 1: Conduct a Hazard Analysis
A hazard is defined as any condition that results in an adverse consequence that is detrimental to the product or to the patient. In HACCP, each part of the

manufacturing process is evaluated to determine whether a particular hazard could result if the step is not controlled. Hazards can be biological (e.g., lack of assurance of sterility for parenterals, objectionable organisms in nonsterile products, endotoxin contamination in excess of the defined limit for parenterals), physical (e.g., nonviable particulate contamination, cracked vials, unseated stoppers), or chemical (e.g., subpotent or super potent drug product).

Principle 2: Identify CCP
Not every action or step, piece of equipment, facility, or utility within a process is critical for each identified hazard. Risk analysis provides a mechanism to scientifically and objectively differentiate points in the process that carry little risk from points that carry considerable risk, and to prioritize these points relative to the identified hazard. Identification of CCPs early in product development identifies a minimum number of important points for initial process validation studies and for routine monitoring, resulting in value-added and efficient process control.

Principle 3: Assign Limits for Each CCP
Each CCP must have an assigned limit that is relevant, accurate, scientifically sound, attainable, and verifiable.

Principle 4: Verify Monitoring and Testing of Limits
Once limits have been assigned, equipment used to take those measurements must be qualified and calibrated, and test methods must be validated.

Principle 5: Verify Corrective Actions
Having a comprehensive process analysis provides the team with the opportunity to anticipate and identify the types of hazard-specific excursions that could happen during routine manufacture, and prospectively analyze each excursion type with regard to its risk to the product and patient. Reasons for excursions can be identified and categorized via a failure mode effect analysis (28) or a similar logic. The HACCP team can then consider and document the types of CAPA that would be appropriate for possible identified failures.

Principle 6: Verify Operational Procedures for CCPs
This step includes writing standard operating procedures (SOPs) and appropriate documentation to identify frequency of routine monitoring, responsibility for data gathering,/analysis/reporting, provisions or out of specification (OOS) investigation, training, preventive maintenance and calibration schemes for equipment.

Principle 7: Verify that Records of Each CCP Are Documented
Process control requires complete and controlled documentation, both for routine release purposes and for diagnostic purposes in the event of a CCP excursion.

APPLYING THE PRINCIPLES OF RISK MANAGEMENT TO THE CONTROL OF ENDOTOXIN CONTAMINATION IN PARENTERALS

Recognizing that cGMPs and the Quality System Regulations are based on the principle of process control, how can a firm utilize the principles of risk analysis to selectively, efficiently, and effectively examine processes and products to understand, anticipate, and minimize the possibility of endotoxin contamination?

Risk management through analysis requires that the entire manufacturing process be objectively examined to identify CCPs. Risk analysis is like peeling an artichoke. Depending on the process or product, risk analyses occur either simultaneously or sequentially on a number of different levels. At the highest levels, the facility, utilities, and systems [e.g., water for injection (WFI), heating, ventilation, and air conditioning (HVAC), cleaning validation and sanitization] are analyzed for the particular hazard, and are validated and monitored according to respective control and CCPs.[a] Once facilities and utilities are analyzed and validated, the risk team can move to the next layer of analysis: the process itself.

On a very high level, one might define CCPs as places in the process where endotoxin can either be added to or eliminated from the system. This can be a daunting task, especially with a complex process, so looking at smaller piece parts makes the analysis process more manageable. In order to study process control, it is most helpful to create a graphic representation the manufacturing process. A map of a simple, generic process is outlined in Figure 1. This process will be the example and reference point for the remainder of this section. For ease of analysis, the process has been divided into five distinct segments:

1. Raw materials: Raw materials/APIs are received into the laboratory for testing against raw-material specifications for disposition by QA.
2. Formulation/compounding: Raw materials and API are formulated in WFI.
3. Filtration: The formulated product is subjected to sterile filtration and then to ultrafiltration immediately prior to filling.
4. Filling: The sterile formulated product is aseptically filled into sterile/depyrogenated vials and stoppered with sterile/depyrogenated closures.
5. End-product testing: The drug product is tested to finished-product specifications for disposition by QA.

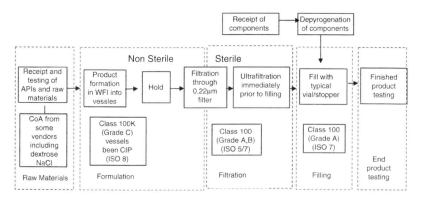

FIGURE 1 Generic process sequence. *Abbreviations*: CIP, clean in place; WFI, water for injection; API, active pharmaceutical ingredient; COA, certificate of analysis.

---

[a] The WFI system, which is a critical system for the control of endotoxin, is discussed in detail in Chapter 7.

For the example, we will make the following assumptions:

- All utilities and systems such as WFI, clean in place (CIP), sterilize in place (SIP), HVAC and cleaning/sanitization have been validated.
- The dose of the example drug product is 1 mL/person and is administered in one single intramuscular (IM) injection/day. This drug has not been approved for use in children.
- The API is chemically synthesized in our facility.
- The active ingredient has a low molecular weight relative to endotoxin aggregates.
- Site audits have not yet been performed for all raw material suppliers.
- Preliminary testing has been performed on a limited number of supplier's pre-shipment samples of raw materials.
- The formulation of the example drug is described in Table 2.

The seven principles of HACCP can applied to the process outlined in Figure 1 as follows:

HACCP Principle 1: Identify the Hazard

For the current discussion, "endotoxin contamination" has been defined as the hazard. Gone untested, undetected, or incorrectly measured, endotoxin contamination can cause serious complications or even the death of a patient receiving adulterated drug product

HACCP Principle 2: Identify CCPs

Each segment of the generic process will be examined objectively for the presence of CCPs. Determination of CCPs must be scientific and unbiased. The consistent use of a decision tree, such as the one outlined in Figure 2, is suggested

Taking each of the five process segments separately, we can use the decision tree to identify CCPs.

Process Segment 1: Raw Materials

"...there was no report that discussed the purity and endotoxin content of raw materials." (FDA 483 citation)

Raw materials come from many sources. Looking across the spectrum of raw materials used in parenteral manufacturing, one might expect that materials

TABLE 2 Formulation of Generic Exemplar Product

Component	Concentration
NaCl	9 (mg/mL)
Dextrose	150 (mg/mL)
Synthesized active pharmaceutical ingredients (drug substance)	75 (mg/mL)
Water for injection	1 mL

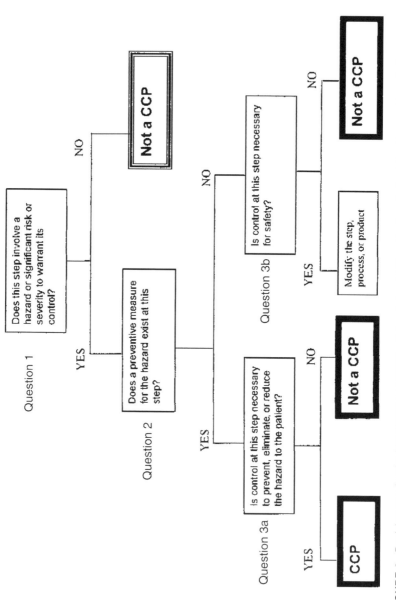

FIGURE 2 Decision tree for the identification of CCPs. *Abbreviation:* CCP, critical control points. *Source:* From Refs. 29 and 31.

isolated from natural sources are likely to contain endotoxin because Gram-negative bacteria are ubiquitous in nature. Components such as sugars and active ingredients such as heparin (extracted and purified from pigs and cows) or active ingredients isolated and purified from fermentations utilizing an *Escherichia coli* host are likely to contain endotoxin (32). Conversely, inorganic salts, strong acids/bases or chemically synthesized materials are less likely to contain endotoxin because the nature of the manufacturing processes are such that they are less subject to contamination by Gram-negative bacteria. Is it acceptable for components of parenteral formulations to contain endotoxin? Yes. The BET cannot measure "0" endotoxin; so material can technically never be labeled as "endotoxin-free" or "pyrogen-free." However, the cumulative level of endotoxin in the particular formulation contributed by individual formulation materials, processing steps, and fill components (vials and stoppers) may not exceed the calculated endotoxin limit for the final drug product. Therefore, without reasonable process control, there is a very real risk that endotoxin in the final product may exceed its calculated endotoxin limit.

Are raw materials CCPs? Raw materials are clearly control points, but their criticality in terms of the potential for endotoxin contamination is dependent on the origin and processing of the raw material and the concentration of the material in the final drug product. The decision tree in Figure 2 was used to document and justify analyses for two common raw materials—dextrose and sodium chloride. Dextrose is derived from corn, and is therefore likely to have some background level of endotoxin. Sodium chloride is an inorganic salt, and as such is less likely to contain endotoxin. Preliminary testing of a number of lots in the laboratory should be performed to confirm any assumptions.

Question 1: Does this step (in this case, this raw material) involve a hazard or significant risk or severity to warrant its control? For dextrose, preliminary testing in the QC laboratory as well as examination of endotoxin test results at our supplier might well reveal that there is considerable lot-to-lot variability in the level of endotoxin in the material. So, the answer for dextrose would be "yes," and we would continue to question no. 2. For sodium chloride, its origin, our vendor audit, the vendor testing, and our preliminary testing might indicate that we find low levels of endotoxin (or perhaps no detectable endotoxin), and that because of the processing of sodium chloride there is no lot-to-lot variability. The answer to question no. 1 for sodium chloride would be "no," and sodium chloride would not be considered to be a critical raw material.

TABLE 3 Decision Tree: Process Segment 1—Raw Materials

	Raw material	
Question	Sodium chloride	Dextrose
1. Does this step involve a hazard or significant risk or severity to warrant its control?	NO (not a CCP)	YES—dextrose is derived from a natural source
2. Does a preventive measure for the hazard exist at this step?	NA	YES—vendor qualification and a CoA will minimize the potential for high levels of endotoxin
3. Is control at this step necessary to prevent, eliminate, or reduce the hazard?		YES—testing of each lot will confirm that endotoxin is below the acceptable limit (CCP)

Abbreviation: CCP, critical control point.

TABLE 4 Decision Tree for Process Segment 2—Formulation

Question	Hold time
1. Does this step involve a hazard or significant risk or severity to warrant its control?	YES—the holding of a nonsterile, formulated drug product could result in bacterial growth. If the growth includes Gram-negative bacteria, the endotoxin levels in the product will increase during the hold time
2. Does a preventive measure for the hazard exist at this step?	YES—validation has confirmed appropriate hold times and temperatures
3. Is control at this step necessary to prevent, eliminate, or reduce the hazard?	YES—if raw materials come in with Gram-negative bioburden or if times and temperatures are not followed, the material could become contaminated with endotoxin that will exceed the depyrogenating ability of our downstream processing

Question 2: Does a preventive measure for the hazard exist at this step? For dextrose, the vendor qualification and initial confirmation of the vendor's certificate of analysis, and the level of dextrose in the finished drug product might provide a level of comfort for the laboratory to accept the CoA in lieu of testing each lot received. So, we will answer "yes" to question no. 2, as we have identified the vendor's processing and testing as a preventive measure.

Question 3a: Is control at this step necessary to prevent, eliminate, or reduce the hazard to the patient? In our case, dextrose is a huge formulation component, and we might feel more comfortable including a QC endotoxin test for each lot received. Our answer to 3a is "yes," so we have now identified dextrose as a CCP.

Another raw material of note is the API. The FDA has repeatedly cited companies for not having endotoxin limits for APIs, indicating that FDA considers the active ingredient to be a critical control point.

> The specification for the active drug substance . . . does not include a microbial content or bacterial endotoxin limit, and the drug substance is not qualified by the vendor from a microbial or bacterial endotoxin perspective. (FDA 483 citation)

Process Segment 2: Formulation
The formulation segment of the process can be subjected to the same decision-making CCP analysis that was used for the raw materials. I have chosen the "hold" step to illustrate the decision process.

> Some batches without established bulk holding times have been held for an extended period of time without bioburden or LAL data to support the time. There was no bioburden or endotoxin testing conducted during validation. (FDA 483 citation)

For our product, raw materials are not sterile and allowing an unpreserved, nonsterile formulation to sit for any appreciable period of time increases the probability of bacterial growth. If any of the bioburden bacteria happen to be Gram negative, this hold step also increases the probability of endotoxin generation. Therefore, because of the variability of numbers and types of microorganisms in the raw materials, the hold step is a CCP even after validation and should be monitored on a routine basis for endotoxin.

If the hold step is on a sterile, formulated product the CCP decision may be very different. Once sterile and held in a sterile container, the bulk should remain sterile. By definition, there are no live Gram-negative bacteria in that solution, so the possibility of proliferation and adding endotoxin during hold time should be non-existent. However, endotoxin testing is an important component of the hold time validation study, to confirm that the combination of vessel, hold time, and hold temperature is not a significant factor.

Process Segment 3: Filtration

Our process specifies two filtrations prior to filling. The first is a filtration through a 0.22 μm filter (sterilizing filter) and the second, immediately prior to filling, is through an ultrafilter (UF), which is intended as a final depyrogenation step. As with any depyrogenating step, the efficiency of the UF in removing endotoxin must be demonstrated (Table 5).

> Review of endotoxin reduction validation studies revealed no control was conducted to determine the amount of endotoxin that can be recovered after seeding the tank with pyrogens. (FDA 483 citation)

The sterilizing filter has no effect on endotoxin. Although the filter is validated for the retention of live and dead bacteria or even larger cell parts, the endotoxin molecule or aggregate is sufficiently small that it will pass through a 0.22 μm filter. Therefore, the sterilizing filter would be a CCP for a different hazard (bioburden or lack of assurance of sterility), but it is not a CCP for the identified endotoxin hazard.

The UF, if sized correctly, will remove endotoxin. UFs are "rated" by the molecular weight of molecules that are retained by the membrane. If the product has a sufficiently low molecular weight as compared to endotoxin, which, depending on aggregation state has a molecular weight of 20,000 to 1,000,000 Da, one can use ultrafiltration to separate endotoxin from formulated product (11–14,33,34). For our example, the UF was deliberately placed in the process after sterile filtration and before filling as a mechanism for depyrogenation. As a depyrogenating device, and as the ultimate step in our process designed specifically for endotoxin removal, the ultrafiltration step is defined as a CCP.

TABLE 5 Decision Tree: Process Segment—Filtration

	Filtration step	
Question	Sterile filtration	Ultrafiltration
1. Does this step involve a hazard or significant risk or severity to warrant its control?	NO. While the sterile filtration might help with the elimination of live Gram-negative bacteria, it will not filter out free endotoxin (not a CCP)	YES—the intent of this step is to remove endotoxin
2. Does a preventive measure for the hazard exist at this step?	NA	Yes—ultrafiltration has been validated
3. Is control at this step necessary to prevent, eliminate, or reduce the hazard?	NA	YES—routine monitoring at this step is important to the control of endotoxin in the final product (CCP)

Abbreviation: CCP, critical control point.

Process Segment 4: Filling
The filling step takes place in a Class 100 (ISO 5) area. Filling needles and filling lines are sterilized. Vials and stoppers are depyrogenated. Although there are many steps in the filling process, we will concentrate on two steps: the depyrogenation of components and the actual filling of the vials (Table 6).

> The firm has not validated the cycle used to depyrogenate vials to ensure proper endotoxin reduction of test vials. (FDA 483 citation)

> The washing process used by the firm for rubber closure components has not been validated for the reduction of endotoxins. (FDA 483 citation)

Incoming Components
Incoming components are not defined in our decision tree as a CCP. As with raw materials, the only way to reduce or eliminate endotoxin at this point is to screen a preshipment sample for endotoxin and reject the lot if the level of endotoxin is found to be in excess of a predetermined limit. Current glass production processes, shrink–wrap packaging, and validated shipping reduce the likelihood of significant contamination, even in nonsterile components. In the case of glass, stoppers, and other components, a subsequent, validated depyrogenation step in the process prior to filling must, by definition, reduce endotoxin by at least three logs to an acceptable level (35). Therefore, while monitoring of incoming components may be useful during validation to determine a baseline for incoming component cleanliness, and while a number of lots might be tested at some interval (perhaps annually) to confirm that endotoxin levels on incoming components are stable and low, we might define incoming components as a control point, rather than a CCP.

TABLE 6 Decision Tree: Process Segment 4—Filling

Question	Filtration step		
	Incoming components	Depyrogenation	Filling
1. Does this step involve a hazard or significant risk or severity to warrant its control?	NO—processing and packaging of components control endotoxin and preliminary testing confirms low, if any, endotoxin is detected (not a CCP)	YES—if not properly validated and if not properly run on a routine basis, components may not be depyrogenated	NO—history of environmental monitoring (including personnel monitoring) does not indicate contamination by Gram-negative bacteria (not a CCP)
2. Does a preventive measure for the hazard exist at this step?	NA	YES—depyrogenation processes have been validated	NA
3. Is control at this step necessary to prevent, eliminate, or reduce the hazard?	NA	YES—continued examination of charts/readouts of depyrogenation procedures must be included in the batch record review process (CCP)	NA

Abbreviation: CCP, critical control point.

Depyrogenation

Depyrogenation processes for vials and stoppers are validated to eliminate or reduce endotoxin to clinically insignificant levels. Per USP, validation of a depyrogenation process requires that at least a three-log reduction be demonstrated from a starting point of at least 1000 recoverable EUs (15,35). Heat-stable components such as glass vials and ampoules and metal instruments are generally depyrogenated by dry heat, while heat-labile components such as rubber stoppers are depyrogenated by long rinsing cycles in WFI. As a terminal depyrogenation step, the depyrogenation process (baking of vials or rinsing of stoppers) is a CCP (see section "Peeling the Artichoke: Determination of CCPs in the Laboratory Performance of the BET Assay" for additional discussion of depyrogenation.).

Filling

The environment is critical to maintaining asepsis during filling. To the extent that control of the environment including air, water, and surfaces eliminates or reduces the probability of introduction and proliferation of *any* microorganism into the environment, it also controls Gram-negatives, and ultimately the potential for endotoxin contamination. Although endotoxin in the air is measured in some environments (e.g., fiber and fabric mills), air in an aseptic area is not routinely monitored for the presence of endotoxin. The possible presence of endotoxin in a classified area is extrapolated from the types and numbers of viable organisms recovered viable air and surface monitoring in the core. Any organism isolated from a Class 100 (ISO 5, EU Grade A/B) environment should be identified to genus and species (23); so the laboratory would be alerted immediately to an outbreak of Gram-negatives in the core.

Fortunately, gram-negative organisms are rarely isolated from a Class 100 aseptic environment. This history suggests that the risk of endotoxin contamination in drug products from normal flora found in aseptic areas is minimal. One estimate for the amount of endotoxin in one *E. coli* cell is 2.9×10^{-4} pg/cell (12). Assuming that the potency of the endotoxin is 10 EU/ng (a common potency for *E. coli* endotoxin), and that the sensitivity of the test system is 0.0625 EU/mL (a common gel clot sensitivity), it would take approximately 21,500 cells/mL to elicit a gel clot positive response. This logic suggests that while environmental control is a CCP for microbial contamination in general, the likelihood of a positive endotoxin result from the environment without a huge and obvious excursion of Gram-negative organisms is minimal. Therefore, we can justifiably call routine environmental control a CCP for asepsis, but a control point for endotoxin.

Although relatively rare, the isolation of a Gram-negative organism in the core is both an out-of-trend excursion and a potential endotoxin generator; so Gram negatives should be treated as objectionable, and their source investigated. Water in the aseptic core, nonvalidated storage of wet components, nonvalidated SIP, or CIP or equipment, and ineffective sanitation/sterilization should be considered when investigating the presence of Gram-negative bacteria in the core or an OOS BET test result. Contact plates from gowning qualification and personnel monitoring must be examined for the presence of Gram-negative bacteria. Operators must undergo training in personal hygiene and aseptic technique to guard against contamination of sterilized/depyrogenated product and components. Operators who show evidence of Gram-negative bacteria either on the gowning qualification or routine personnel monitoring samples, or operators who are ill must be reassigned to tasks outside of the core until investigation and/or retraining is completed.

Process Segment 5: Finished Product Testing

The final step in our generic process is finished-product testing. As with sterility, the state called "free of detectable endotoxin" cannot be assured through finished product testing—it is assured through careful process validation and value-added monitoring for routine process control. If a process is validated and is in control, the result of the finished-product testing should be a foregone conclusion.

The FDA Guideline for Limulus Amebocyte Lysate (LAL) testing of finished products requires that a minimum of three units, representing the beginning, middle, and end of the fill be tested for endotoxin. For medical devices, the minimum number of units selected for testing is dependent on the lot size (6). The harmonized pharmacopeial chapters are silent on the issue of sampling.

Although the number of test units is statistically insignificant, the results of finished product testing are extremely important. An OOS result on any one of the individual units or on the pool of the units culled at random from across the filling run can cause the entire batch to be rejected unless contamination during testing, a breach of the test protocol that could have resulted in a false positive, operator error, contaminated test equipment, or the use of inappropriate reagents can be unequivocally demonstrated and documented (36). As with the sterility test, it is imperative in BET testing that the assay be kept as clean as possible to avoid the possibility of a false positive. Qualified analysts who can demonstrate good aseptic technique, equipment that is clean and free of detectable endotoxin, a validated test method and qualified/calibrated assay equipment are all vital prerequisites to a valid BET test (Table 7).

Thus, the performance of test itself, including the reagents, the equipment, the method, and the analyst is a critical control step in any process employing the BET. For a more detailed analysis of test methodology, see section "Peeling the Artichoke: Determination of CCPs in the Laboratory Performance of the BET Assay."

Many segments in our generic process could require additional, more task-specific risk analyses. For example, the following task-specific processes should be further examined for the presence of CCPs for the endotoxin hazard:

- The synthesis or fermentation process for our API
- Any depyrogenation step (section "Peeling the Artichoke: Determination of CCPs in the Laboratory Performance of the BET Assay")
- The testing process itself (section "Peeling the Artichoke: Determination of CCPs in the Laboratory Performance of the BET Assay")

TABLE 7 Decision Tree: Process Segment 5—Testing

Question	Finished product testing
1. Does this step involve a hazard or significant risk or severity to warrant its control?	YES—there is a significant risk of a false result if the bacterial endotoxins test is not validated or if it is improperly performed
2. Does a preventive measure for the hazard exist at this step?	YES—analyst qualification, reagent confirmation of label claim (or standard curve linearity), product validation, and routine system suitability all provide assurance that the test is performing correctly
3. Is control at this step necessary to prevent, eliminate, or reduce the hazard?	YES—the test and its accessories must be continually controlled to assure a valid test result (CCP)

Abbreviation: CCP, critical control point.

■ Complex formulations
■ Labor-intensive or equipment-intensive manufacturing steps

Control points and CCPs for our generic process as identified in HACCP Principle 2 are summarized in Table 8.

HACCP Principle 3: Assigning Endotoxin Limits

Once CCPs have been identified, scientifically sound and attainable endotoxin limits must be assigned. Initially, action limits are calculated and assigned for the drug product and to all critical materials and processing steps. As process experience is gained, action limits may be modified and alert limits may be set based on historical data and process capability, recognizing possible seasonal fluctuations in the endotoxin content of incoming city water and raw materials.

> Endotoxins were not evaluated during validation and there was not data to justify established endotoxin specifications. (FDA 483 citation)

The calculated endotoxin limit for a drug product is the maximum allowable level of endotoxin for a product with a specific formula and an identified maximum dose per kilogram patient weight, route of administration length of administration. For endotoxin testing, compendial limits exist for drug products and WFI, but not for raw materials, individual APIs, and formulation excipients (18,20). In order to assign limits to items for which no published limit exists, we must start with the calculated limit for the finished drug product and work backward to "distribute" the allowable endotoxin among the various formulation components. Any assumptions that are made during this exercise must be clearly stated, explained, and justified.

Calculating Endotoxin Limits for Small-Volume Parenteral Drug Products

The endotoxin limit for a SVP drug product is defined on the basis of dose, and is calculated using the following formula:

$$\text{Endotoxin limit} = \frac{K}{M}$$

where K is the threshold human pyrogenic dose (5.0 EU/kg for any route of administration other than intrathecal, 0.2 EU/kg for those drug products administered

TABLE 8 Summary of Control and Critical Control Points for the Process Outlined in Figure 1

	Identified control point	Manufacturing segment
Uncontrolled points	Sterile filtration	Filtration
Control points	Sodium chloride	Raw materials
	Incoming components	Filling
	Filling environment	Filling
Critical control points	Active pharmaceutical ingredient	Raw materials
	Dextrose	Raw materials
	Holding of formulated product	Formulation
	Ultrafiltration	Filtration
	Depyrogenation	Filling
	Drug-product testing	Laboratory testing

intrathecally), M is the maximum recommended human dose of product/kg of body weight administered in a single one-hour period.

For our example, the dose of the product is 1 mL/person, and our drug is administered in a single IM injection (assumptions and Table 2). We assume that the average person weighs 70 kg (3,6,37). Therefore, the total allowable endotoxin per person would be the following:

70 kg/person $\times$ 5EU/kg = 350 EU/person

The endotoxin limit for our product is calculated as follows:

$$\text{Limit} = \frac{K}{M} = \frac{5.0 \text{ EU/kg}}{1.0 \text{ mL/70 kg}} = 350 \text{ EU/mL}$$

Therefore, the maximum level of endotoxin "available" to us for distribution among all components in the formulation, including stoppers and vials, is 350 EU/mL (Fig. 3).

The endotoxin limit specification for a drug product may not exceed this calculated value, but a firm may choose to assign a lower, more stringent endotoxin limit for the product. This lower limit provides manufacturers with a "safety factor" and can be justified given the follows:

■ The patient could be on multiple therapies, each of which can potentially contribute endotoxin. We tend to think of the endotoxin limit in terms of only one therapy per patient, but we must realize that the 5 EU/kg limit is really the sum of all endotoxin sources. Thus, it is in the patient's best interest that the detectable endotoxin in any one-drug product be well below the allowable limit.
■ The BET has a considerable error (see section "Segment 5: Data Analysis and Interpretation").

Often, firms choose half or quarter of the calculated endotoxin limit as their in-house specification for a well-characterized product and process. Although manufacturing a product with very low endotoxin is clearly in the patient's interest, there are some cautionary notes on the practice of assigning "safety factor" in-house endotoxin limits.

■ If the in-house final product specification is lower than the calculated or compendial limit, a product may not be released if it fails the in-house specification but passes the compendial or calculated specification. Therefore, if the in-house limit is set too low, product may be rejected unnecessarily.
■ In-house limits that are different than calculated limits must be set relative to the documented manufacturing history of the product (process capability) rather than an arbitrary or common level. Setting endotoxin limits without

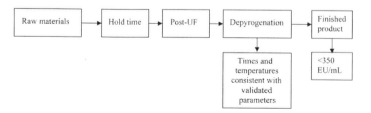

FIGURE 3 Assigning limits relative to process flow: drug product. *Abbreviations*: EU, endotoxin unit; UF, ultrafilter.

any supporting manufacturing data might result in a number of unnecessary excursions, investigations, and rejected lots of product.

■ Validation activities must reference either the calculated limit or the in-house specification whichever is lower.

■ In-house limits must be set carefully. Once a more stringent in-house limit is set, it is very difficult to justify increasing it back to the calculated limit.

Until some experience is gained with the product and process, it is advisable to set the in-house limit for the drug product at the calculated endotoxin limit for the product. In our example, the limit would be 350 EU/mL (calculated above). This calculation satisfies the requirement to put a limit on the finished product test.

Calculating Endotoxin Limits for Identified CCPs

We can now work backward through the process to calculate limits for in-process samples, noncompendial materials, and compendial materials with no published limits (Figs. 4–7).

The depyrogenation of components (vials, stoppers) had been identified by the decision tree as a critical processing step. The most sensitive, generally available gel-clot reagent has a label claim sensitivity of 0.03125 EU/mL. The limit of quantitation (LOQ) for the photometric tests can be as low as 0.001 EU/mL, but more often than not, the LOQ is 0.005 EU/mL. However, we want our vials to be free of any detectable endotoxin, and we know from our validation studies that we get at least a three-log reduction from the depyrogenation process. For a dry heat depyrogenation step or for a validated rinsing step, attention to the validated time/temperature parameters during manufacturing and the checking of times/temperatures during batch record review will tell us more about the effectiveness of a depyrogenation process than a negative test on an empty vial or stopper. Even though depyrogenation is a CCP, our routine limit will not be a specific endotoxin test on depyrogenated vials, but rather confirmation during batch record review that the time/temperature of the depyrogenation process as documented meets the validation specifications for the load.

Clearly, we want to make sure that the product downstream of the UF (post-UF), meets the endotoxin specification for the final product. An argument could be made to set the limit for the "postultrafiltration" at the calculated limit for the product, but it would be more prudent to set the limit incrementally lower, given that there are activities and components (vials, stoppers) that come into contact with the product postultrafiltration. Assuming that we have validation data on UF efficiency, it is reasonable to set the post-UF limit at less than half of the drug-product limit. After

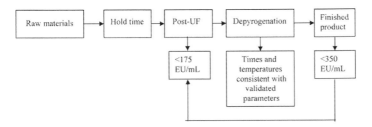

FIGURE 4 Assigning endotoxin limits relative to process flow: depyrogenation. *Abbreviations*: EU, endotoxin unit; UF, ultrafilter.

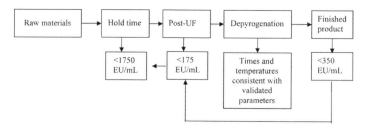

FIGURE 5 Assigning endotoxin limits relative to process flow: post-UF. *Abbreviations*: EU, endo-toxin unit; UF, ultrafilter.

collecting sufficient historical data on this step, we may choose to tighten the limit to align with process capability. Setting this limit lower than the drug-product limit should help assure that the drug product, in the absence of testing error or overt contamination event in filling, will *always* meet the specification.

If we work back through the process one more step, we can assign an endo-toxin limit to the formulated bulk posthold and upstream of the ultrafiltration (preaseptic filtration and pre-UF). This hold is on nonsterile, formulated bulk, which poses some unique considerations. The limit that we assign must depend on the following:

- The history of the endotoxin levels and bioburden levels in the formulated bulk upstream of the sterilizing filter (e.g., are Gram-negatives normally isolated from the prefiltration bulk bioburden samples?),
- The efficiency of the UF to remove endotoxin, which is demonstrated during the validation of the process, and
- Validation data from the hold time studies.

In the absence of historical data, but recognizing the validated ability of the UF to provide a three-log reduction in endotoxin, we could justifiably set a limit for the unfiltered bulk that is an order of magnitude higher than the downstream limit. Therefore, we might allow no more than 1750 EU/mL upstream of the UF. Again, once we gain experience with quantitative and qualitative bioburden and endotoxin in the formulated product at the end of the holding time, we could easily adjust this limit. A second check on this CCP is at the batch record

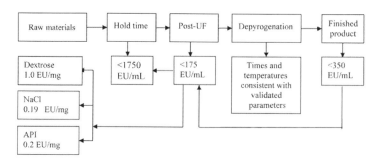

FIGURE 6 Assigning endotoxin limits relative to process flow ultrafiltration. *Abbreviations*: EU, endotoxin unit; UF, ultrafilter.

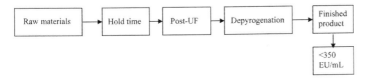

FIGURE 7 Assigning endotoxin limits relative to process flow: raw materials. *Abbreviations*: EU, endotoxin unit; UF, ultrafilter.

review stage, where the reviewer will confirm that the actual hold time did not exceed the validated limit. However, assuming that a validated three-log reduction in product stream endotoxin has been validated for the UF, we should detect less than 1.7 EU/mL downstream of the UF—two orders of magnitude lower than specified, and providing an additional safety factor for our drug product.

Assigning limits to noncompendial items such as raw materials and excipients can be complicated. The simple formulation for our drug product is outlined in Table 2. As there is the possibility of further contamination during filling, we will work backwards from the post-UF sample limit of <175 EU/mL rather than the drug product limit of <350 EU/mL to assign limits to individual components.

There are a number of thought processes that might be used in order to distribute the allowable endotoxin of 175 EU/mL:

Method 1: We have four components in our formulation. If we assume that each component of the formulation is allowed to contribute 25% of the allowable endotoxin load, our calculated endotoxin limits, corrected for component concentration in the final drug product, would be as in Table 9. There are a number of troubling issues with this scenario:

- Our allowable limit for WFI far exceeds the compendial limit of not more than 0.25 EU/mL.
- Dextrose, the raw material that is likely to contribute the most endotoxin to our formulation, is allowed the least amount of endotoxin per unit weight.
- Sodium chloride, a raw material that is not likely to contribute significant endotoxin to our final product, is given a limit that is an order of magnitude higher than the either the API or the dextrose.

Method 2: We can assign an endotoxin limit[b] to all of the ingredients equally per unit of weight. If we add up all of the ingredients, we have 234 mg of dry ingredients in the formulation. If we assume that the contribution of the WFI is negligible relative to the limit we have set or the product (the WFI compendial limit of not more than 0.25 EU/mL relative to our assigned limit of 175 EU/mL), we can equally divide our 175 EU among the 234 mg in the formulation:

$$\frac{175 \text{ EU/mL}}{234 \text{ mg/mL}} = 0.74 \text{ EU/mg}$$

By this method, each milligram of material in the formulation, regardless of origin, would be allowed to contribute 0.74 EU. Although these numbers seem to be more reasonable than the limits calculated in method 1, there is still a problem with this method in that we have assigned the same limit to the raw material that is

---

[b] When rounding endotoxin limits, it is prudent to round all calculated endotoxin limits down to the more conservative number.

TABLE 9 Calculation of Endotoxin Limits for Formulation Components: Method 1

Component	EU/mL	Concentration (mg/mL)	Calculated endotoxin level
NaCl	43.75	9	4.86 EU/mg
Dextrose	43.75	150	0.291 EU/mg
Active pharmaceutical ingredient	43.75	75	0.583 EU/mg
Water for injection	43.75	1 mL	43.75 EU/mL

Abbreviation: EU, endotoxin unit.

most likely to contribute endotoxin (dextrose) as to the raw material that is least likely to contribute endotoxin (sodium chloride or our synthesized API).

Method 3: We can assign endotoxin limits based on the percentage of the material in the final formulation, assuming that the WFI contribution is negligible, for our example (Table 10).

Working through the calculation, we find that if we assign an endotoxin limit for each component based on percentage in the final formulation and then adjust for the concentrations of each component, we get the same result as in Method 2, and we are left with the same concerns as for Method 2.

Method 4: We can allocate endotoxin based on the source of the raw material. For this method, we will need to clearly articulate and document our assumptions:

- Contribution by WFI is negligible at below 0.25 EU/mL.
- Dextrose is the only component in the formulation from a natural source; so it can be assumed that it will be the most variable in endotoxin content and the most likely to contribute endotoxin to the final product. Preliminary testing has confirmed that endotoxin in incoming dextrose is quite variable. In the example, we have allowed the dextrose to contribute 90% of the total allowable endotoxin in the formulation.
- Sodium chloride is an inorganic salt and is not likely to contribute large amounts of endotoxin to our product. Preliminary testing of a number of lots of sodium chloride has confirmed that endotoxin levels are consistently low. In the example, we limit sodium chloride to 1% of the total allowable endotoxin.
- The API is the product of a chemical synthesis and as such, has a low probability of contributing endotoxin contamination relative to the dextrose. We have allowed it to contribute 9% of the drug product limit.

Given these assumptions, we might assign endotoxin limits that are somewhat arbitrary, but are based on a logic that is supported by preliminary testing data (Table 11).

Using this method, we have shifted the bulk of the allowable endotoxin (90%) to the component that is most likely to contribute endotoxin—the dextrose.

TABLE 10 Calculation of Endotoxin Limits for Formulation Components: Method 3

Component	Concentration (mg/mL)	Percentage of formulation	EU/mL	EU/mg
NaCl	9	38	6.65	0.74
Dextrose	150	64	112	0.74
Active pharmaceutical ingredient	75	32	56	0.74

Abbreviation: EU, endotoxin unit.

TABLE 11 Calculation of Endotoxin Limits for Formulation Components: Method 4

Component	Assigned percentage total EU	EU/mL	Concentration (mg/mL)	EU/mg
NaCl	1	1.75	9	0.19
Dextrose	90	157.5	150	1.05
Active pharmaceutical ingredient	9	15.75	75	0.21

Abbreviation: EU, endotoxin unit.

By this method, we have allowed the dextrose to contribute about 50% more endotoxin than any of the other three methods for assigning limits to raw materials (above), and we have allowed the dextrose to contribute endotoxin at a level that is at least five times higher than any other formulation component[c].

Out of the four methods, Method 4 provides the most flexibility in assigning endotoxin limits to the components of any given formulation. However, we cannot create a circumstance where the same raw material could have different endotoxin limits depending on the formulation in which it is used. To standardize limits and make laboratory testing easier, we need to choose the most stringent of the endotoxin limits that have been calculated for any raw material across the company's product line. An example in Table 12 illustrates endotoxin limits for three different fictitious formulations.

For example, sodium chloride is used in all three of the formulations, but the most stringent limit is 0.001 EU/mg that has been assigned for Formulation B. If we make this limit our company specification for NaCl, we will be assured that the raw material will also meet the requirements for Formulations A and C. The company-wide, rounded down specifications for these raw materials in Table 12 would be:

- Dextrose: 1.0 EU/mg
- NaCl: 0.001 EU/mg
- Sodium phosphate monobasic: 0.03 EU/mg
- Mannitol: 0.5 EU/mg.

Tabulating and choosing endotoxin limits in this way accomplishes two things:

- It makes laboratory testing more efficient in that all lots of raw material, regardless of the final formulation, are tested against a single specification.

TABLE 12 Choosing Endotoxin Limits

Material	Formulation A: EU/mg (our example, Table 2)	Formulation B: EU/mg	Formulation C: EU/mg
NaCl	1.75	0.001	0.4
Dextrose	1.05	2.0	N/A
Sodium phosphate monobasic	N/A	0.35	0.03
Mannitol	N/A	N/A	0.53

Abbreviations: EU, endotoxin unit; N/A, not applicable.

---

[c] If the formulation contained multiple components from natural sources or if the API were the product of fermentation, we might think differently and distribute our endotoxin using a different set of assumptions that are more appropriate to the formulation. The only requirement of method 4 is that assumptions are clearly articulated, justified, and documented.

■ Because the most stringent formulation is chosen for the specification, the firm can be assured that no raw material will contribute endotoxin to a formulation in excess of its allowable limit

In summary, controls and limits can be assigned to identified CCPs as in Table 13.

HACCP Principle 4: Verify Monitoring and Testing of Limits

HACCP Principle 4 requires that limits are valid and that the test methods and equipment used to measure endotoxin are also validated/qualified. For any CCP requiring a BET, the test method would be validated according to the harmonized pharmacopeia and the FDA Guideline (3–6). Any valid BET assay requires the following prerequisite tests:

■ Analysts must be qualified (6).
■ The lysate reagent label claim or standard curve linearity must be verified (3–6).
■ If a secondary endotoxin standard [control standard endotoxin (CSE)] is used for the assay, it must be compared and standardized against the primary endotoxin standard [reference standard endotoxin (RSE)] for every unique combination of CSE lot/lysate lot used in the laboratory (6).
■ The consumable equipment must be shown to be free of interference and detectable endotoxin (3–5).

TABLE 13 Summary of Control and Critical Control Points for the Process Outlined in Figure 1

Identified critical control point	Manufacturing segment	Sample to be tested or document to be examined	Limit	Responsibility
Dextrose	Raw materials	Dextrose	<1.0 EU/mg	Quality control testing
Active pharmaceutical ingredient	Raw materials	Active pharmaceutical ingredient	<0.2 EU/mg	Quality control testing
Holding of formulated product		Posthold/ preultrafilter	<1750 EU/mL	Quality control testing
		Batch record	Hold time not to exceed specified limits	Manufacturing; quality assurance batch record review
Ultrafiltration	Filtration	Postultrafilter	<175 EU/mL	Quality control testing
Depyrogenation	Filling	Batch record	Conformance to validated time/temperature	Manufacturing; quality assurance batch record reviews
Drug product testing	Laboratory	Filled vials	<350 EU/mL	Quality control testing

Abbreviation: EU, endotoxin unit.

- Laboratory equipment used in the performance of the BET including pipettors, depyrogenation ovens, incubating devices, mixers, and photometric readers must be calibrated/qualified/validated as appropriate. Software used in the calculation, tabulation, and trending of endotoxin test data must be validated and must be 21 CFR Part 11 compliant (Table 14).

HACCP Principle 5: Verify Corrective and Preventive Actions

Prior to implementing a HACCP plan, possible failure scenarios should be anticipated and identified so that appropriate CAPAs can be defined ahead of time and implemented quickly if needed. This exercise serves two purposes: (*i*) It provides the opportunity for objective analysis of possible failure without the stress of a pending investigation and (*ii*) it provides the opportunity for the definition of unbiased and scientifically supported CAPAs that can be uniformly applied to all similar excursions going forward.

For example, the vial depyrogenation process, which has been identified as a CCP, might fail to meet the time/temperature parameters determined in the validation study and required by the batch record. Possible reasons and associated CAPAs for this failure might include those shown in Table 15.

HACCP Principle 6: Verify Operational Procedures

Once process validation is complete, implementation of routine testing requires that the proper infrastructure is in place. Training of new operators and analysts

TABLE 14 Hazard and Critical Control Point Analysis Principle 4: Verification of Monitoring and Testing for Endotoxin[a]

Identified critical control point	Laboratory SOPs	Equipment/systems to be qualified	Validation protocols and reports
Dextrose, active pharmaceutical ingredient	Testing SOP	Testing equipment[b]	BET test method for the raw material
Holding of formulated product		Testing equipment	BET test method for the process intermediate
Ultrafiltration	Testing SOP	UF removal efficiency	BET test method for the process intermediate
		Testing equipment	UF endotoxin removal efficiency
Depyrogenation	Preparation and use of endotoxin indicators for depyrogenation studies	Depyrogenation oven (heat stable items) Washing machine (heat labile items) Testing equipment	Depyrogenation parameters for identified load patterns (time/temperature)
Drug product testing	Testing SOP	Testing equipment	BET test method for the drug product

[a]Over and above the prerequisite testing described above.
[b]Testing equipment includes pipettes, tubes, pipettors, heat blocks/water baths for gel clot testing; pipettes, tubes, pipettors, plates, plate/tube reader, and data analysis software for photometric tests.
Abbreviations: SOP, standard operating procedure; CIP, clean in place; BET, bacterial endotoxins; UF, ultrafilter; SIP, sterilize in place.

TABLE 15 Analysis of a Possible Depyrogenation Failure[a]

Failure mode	Potential effects	Potential causes of failure	Detection method	Recommended action
Incomplete cycle (failure to meet time/tempera-ture requirements)	Inefficient depyrogenation could result in vials contaminated with endotoxin, and therefore drug product contaminated with endotoxin	Power failure Equipment failure (timer, tempera-ture controller, chart recorder) Operator failure to set proper time/ temperature parameters	Alarm, building management system, or chart recorder Chart recorder/ BMS record review Chart recorder/ BMS record review	Provide back-up power to depyrogenation equipment Increased attention to or frequency of preventive maintenance, calibration Retraining

[a]After failure modes and effects analysis.
Source: From Ref. 30.
Abbreviation: BMS, building management system.

and retraining of veteran employees should be consistent, repeated at defined intervals, and well documented. Validation, calibration and qualification philoso-phies, and strategies should be clearly articulated in master plans that reference appropriate in-house specifications as well as regulatory, compliance, and industry-consensus documents. Strategies and methods should be harmonized where possible among laboratories, processing areas, and manufacturing sites so that data from similar or identical processes are comparable. Equipment must be requalified and recalibrated according to manufacturer's instructions and/or a defined calibration schedule. For example:

- Depyrogenation ovens should always be requalified upon the introduction of a novel load pattern, but must be requalified at least annually.
- Changes to processes may require revalidation as determined by change control.
- Control may also require BET revalidation of raw materials as part of the quali-fication of a second supplier.

HACCP Principle 7: Verification of Documentation
The following documents are necessary components of a complete drug product batch record or device history record. These documents must reflect routine moni-toring for all CCPs.

- Comprehensive, complete, reviewed, and signed batch records including manufacturing processes and QC testing
- Change control for processes, facilities, testing, or software
- Approved variances or deviations for manufacturing or testing
- Approved investigations for excursions and product OOS results

PEELING THE ARTICHOKE: DETERMINATION OF CCPs IN THE LABORATORY PERFORMANCE OF THE BET ASSAY
Laboratory testing has been identified by the decision tree as a CCP (Table 7). We can "peel the artichoke" and examine the sequence of events in the laboratory testing

segment using much the same thought process as we looked at the sequence of steps in the generic aseptic manufacturing process (above). How do we define control points and CCPs in the test procedure? The new hazard for laboratory testing is "false test results." The task is to identify those steps in the testing process that can be primarily responsible for the generation of "false" results—either false positives (a significant compliance and financial issue for the company) or false negatives (a significant safety hazard to the patient and a compliance as well as legal issue for the firm).

Bacterial Endotoxins Test Methodologies

Three technologies are described in the pharmacopeia for use in the performance of the BET. All three use a reagent that is formulated from the blood of the horseshoe crab. The reagent is called LAL. *Limulus* is the genus name of the North-American horseshoe crab, *Limulus polyphemus*; Amebocyte is the name of the circulating blood cells of the horseshoe crab; and Lysate describes the disruption of the amebocytes, which is a step in the preparation of the reagent. Lysate can also be made from the blood of the Asian horseshoe crab, *Tachepleyus tridentatus*. This lysate is called TAL. For a more complete and detailed discussion of BET reagents and methodologies, see Ref. 11.

The Gel Clot Test

In nature, the horseshoe crab's blood clots as part of an immune response to the presence of endotoxin. The gel-clot test is an in vitro test based on the in vivo reaction of the blood of the horseshoe crab with endotoxin. The presence of endotoxin, through a cascade of reactions, results in the cleaving of the coagulogen molecule (the clotting protein) to create a peptide called coagulin. The more the endotoxin at the beginning of the cascade, the more the coagulin at the end. If enough coagulin molecules are generated, they form a matrix that is visually observed as a clot. The sensitivity of the gel-clot reagent defines the limit of detection of the test system. Thus, if a reagent is labeled with a sensitivity of 0.0625 EU/mL, it means that the reagent will clot in the presence of 0.0625 EU/mL or more of endotoxin in a noninterfering test solution.

The gel-clot test is binary. If, upon 180° inversion, the clot remains at the bottom of the tube, the test is positive. Any other reaction is scored as a negative. Two types of gel-clot tests are described in the pharmacopeia: the limits test and the assay. The limits test is a qualitative test, where a single dilution of the test sample is assayed, and the result is reported as "$< \lambda$ EU/mL" or "$\geq \lambda$ EU/mL" where λ is the confirmed label claim sensitivity of the reagent. For example, if a WFI sample is tested using lysate where $\lambda = 0.125$ EU/mL, and the result is observed and scored as negative, the endotoxin level in the sample is reported as less than 0.125 EU/mL. If the sample induces a gel, the sample is scored as positive, and the result is reported as 0.125 EU/mL or above. If a sample must be diluted for the test, the result is reported as $< (\lambda)$(dilution factor) mL or $\geq (\lambda)$(dilution factor mL).

The assay is a more quantitative gel-clot test. For the assay, the test sample is diluted, and each dilution is tested using the gel-clot method. The last tube in the dilution series that scores positive and is followed by a negative response is called the endpoint dilution. Endotoxin content in a gel-clot assay is calculated and reported as equal to the (endpoint dilution factor) (λ). For example, if the endpoint in a dilution series of city water is 1:250 and λ is equal to 0.125 EU/mL, the result is calculated and reported as:

$$\begin{aligned}
\text{Endotoxin level} &= (\text{endpoint dilution factor})(\lambda)\\
&= (250)(0.125\,\text{EU/mL})\\
&= 31.25\,\text{EU/mL}
\end{aligned}$$

Photometric Tests

Although the gel-clot test is capable of producing a quantitative result, the assay is labor-intensive and time-consuming. The photometric tests are based on the work performed by Drs. Jack Levin and Frederick Bang who, in 1968, reported on the kinetics of the reaction between lysate and endotoxin. Levin and Bang (38) looked at the kinetics of the lysate reaction by measuring the optical density (i.e., accumulation of coagulin) over time after the addition of endotoxin. Figure 8 is a representation of the kinetic reactions of a series of endotoxin standards.

They made two important observations: (i) that the higher the endotoxin concentration, the shorter the "lag" time (i.e., the part at the initiation of the reaction where no observable change in optical density takes place), and (ii) the higher the endotoxin concentration, the faster the rate of the reaction, once initiated. These observations form the foundation of the two basic photometric methods: the endpoint and the kinetic assays. In the photometric assays, endotoxin standards prepared in LAL reagent water (LRW) are used to construct the standard curve.

Two of the photometric assays use a synthetic substrate as a substitute for the coagulogen molecule. A chromophore is coupled to the substrate so that in the absence of an activated clotting enzyme, the solution containing the substrate–chromophore complex is clear. When the clotting enzyme is activated by endotoxin, the chromophore is cleared from the substrate. The cleaved chromophore is yellow. As with coagulin, the rate of formation of yellow color is proportional to the level of activated clotting enzyme, which in turn is proportional to the level of endotoxin that is present in the system.

Endpoint chromogenic assay: In the endpoint chromogenic assay, the LAL reaction is stopped at a point in time (dotted line, Fig. 9A) by the addition of acetic acid, which freezes the color formation. Software prepares a standard curve of the intensity of the yellow color as a function of the endotoxin concentration. The result is a linear standard curve with a positive slope (a direct relationship between color

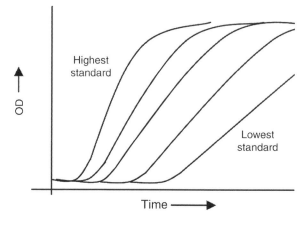

FIGURE 8 Kinetics of the limulus amebocyte lysate (LAL) reaction. *Source*: From Ref. 38. *Abbreviation*: OD, optical density.

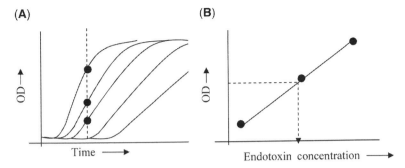

FIGURE 9 Endpoint chromogenic assay (**A**) and standard curve (**B**). *Abbreviation*: OD, optical density.

intensity and endotoxin concentration), and a range of about one log (Fig. 9A). The yellow color formed in unknowns is similarly "frozen," and the endotoxin content is determined by interpolation from the standard curve (dotted line, Figure 9b).

Kinetic assay: The major limitation of the endpoint chromogenic assay is that the standard curve range is limited to about one log. One may look at the same set of endotoxin standards and ask a different question: How long does it take for each standard to reach a targeted optical density? The dotted line in Figure 10A represents the "onset" or "reaction" optical density. The assay measures the time that it takes for each standard and sample to reach the onset OD. The standard curve is constructed by plotting the log of the onset time as a function of the log of the endotoxin concentration (Fig. 10B). Data transformation is necessary to construct a linear standard curve. The relationship between onset time and endotoxin concentration is an inverse one. "Lower" endotoxin concentrations take a "longer" time to reach the onset OD.

The Testing Sequence
Following the logic stream used for the analysis of the manufacturing process, the testing sequence can be divided into four testing segments: initial QC, validation, routine testing, data analysis, and interpretation (Fig. 11). We can identify test

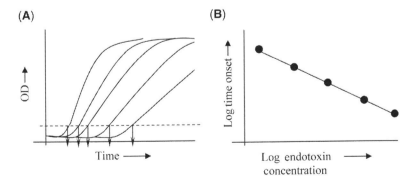

FIGURE 10 Kinetic assay (**A**) and standard curve (**B**). *Abbreviation*: OD, optical density.

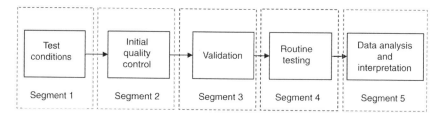

FIGURE 11 Generic bacterial endotoxins testing sequence.

controls or prerequisites in each of these segments, which will help us understand the criticality of the assay. To simplify this analysis, let us make the following assumptions:

■ Training and appropriate SOPs are critical to any operation, and by definition are CCPs. For the example, let us assume that SOPs are in place and training has been successfully completed.
■ All equipment has been properly qualified and documented.

Segment 1: Test Conditions
The segment defined as "test conditions" is a catch-all to describe the basic environment for performing the test (Fig. 12). Two major areas are examined in this category, although more might be defined in a particular laboratory setting. The conditions that have been chosen for this example that could adversely affect the test and result in false results are analyst technique, and test area cleanliness classification (i.e., Class 100, Class 10,000, etc.).

Technique
Any BET is technique dependent. Literature and logic tell us that it takes a large number of Gram-negative organisms to cause a false positive in an LAL test. While these large numbers are not generally contributed solely by the room air, they could potentially be contributed by poor aseptic technique during the testing of small volume samples. For example, touching the "working end" of the pipette, getting fingers inside the reaction tubes, and poor pipetting technique, which could result in endotoxin carryover, can result in a false positive result. Any positive is considered to be a de facto product failure unless it can be proven and documented that the result is the product of poor technique (36). Likewise, improper dilution of a drug product that interferes with the test could result in a false negative. Improper "spiking" of positive controls could result in a voided test. Unless someone is watching the operator at all times, poor technique is

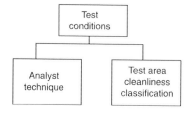

FIGURE 12 Test conditions.

difficult to prove, meaning that false positive tests often, if not regularly, result in unnecessary product rejection. Thus, proper technique certainly reduces the possibility of a false result, and therefore it is a "critical control factor" in the performance of the BET.

Room Air Classification

It takes a large number of Gram-negative bacteria from the air to cause a false result in a BET. Sample preparation may be performed in a laminar flow hood as added protection against contamination, but because the test is incubated uncovered out on the bench, the use of laminar flow hood is not a necessary precaution, particularly if the analyst is skilled in aseptic technique. There is one notable exception, however. If the sample is potentially toxic or harmful to the analyst, it should be prepared in a biosafety cabinet (BSC) and under conditions that protect the person. A clean and tidy laboratory environment consistent with 21 CFR 211, "cGMP for Finished Pharmaceuticals" and 21 CFR 58, "Good Laboratory Practices for nonclinical laboratory studies" is all that is needed to run the BET (7,9). Therefore, the room's cleanliness classification (i.e., Class 100, Class 10,000) is not a critical control factor.

Segment 2: Initial Quality Control

The initial QC segment of the process identifies all the prerequisites necessary prior to running a valid routine test. In total, these activities demonstrate that the laboratory, including analysts, reagents, environment, equipment, and test methods are "in control." "All of the requirements of initial QC are listed in either the harmonized pharmacopeial chapters, the lysate manufacturer's product inserts, or the 1987 FDA Guideline. Therefore they are, by default, CCPs in the performance of the BET" (Lysate manufacturers' product inserts) (3–6). Prerequisites are shown in Figure 13.

Lysate Label Claim/Linearity Verification

The sensitivity of each lot of lysate reagent is initially determined by the manufacturer and is then confirmed and certified by FDA's Center for Biologics Evaluation and Research (CBER) before release for sale (3–6). The 1987 FDA Guideline and all of the current pharmacopeia state that the sensitivity of each new lot of lysate reagent that is received in the laboratory must be confirmed by the laboratory before use. The idea is *not* to reassign sensitivity to the reagent, but rather to

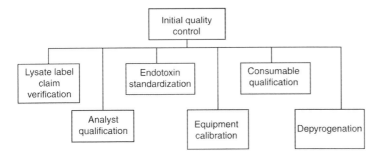

FIGURE 13 Prerequisites (initial quality control) to the bacterial endotoxins test.

demonstrate that the testing laboratory can replicate the result obtained both by the lysate manufacturer and by the CBER.

For gel clot, an endotoxin standard is diluted in LAL reagent water (LRW) to "bracket" the label claim sensitivity of the reagent. Bracket means diluting the endotoxin standard to concentrations equal to 2λ, λ, $\frac{1}{2}\lambda$, and $\frac{1}{4}\lambda$, where λ is the label claim sensitivity of the reagent. These four endotoxin dilutions are tested in quadruplicate, and the endpoints (i.e., last positive test result followed by a negative result) for each of the four replicate series is determined. Because the dilution series is geometric rather than arithmetic, the determined lysate sensitivity is calculated using a geometric mean:

$$GM = antilog\left(\frac{\Sigma \log_{10} \text{endpoint}}{f}\right)$$

where f is the number of replicates.

Table 16 is an example of a gel clot label claim verification study. In this case, λ is 0.125 EU/mL. The geometric mean for this example is calculated as follows:

$$GM = antilog\left(\frac{-0.903 + -1.204 + -1.204 + -0.903}{4}\right)$$
$$= antilog(-1.0535) = 0.088\ EU/mL$$

The lysate label claim sensitivity is confirmed if the geometric mean of the replicate endpoints is equal to the label claim ± one twofold dilution (i.e., within the window of 2λ to $\frac{1}{2}\lambda$). In the example, the determined label claim is 0.088 EU/mL, which is within the window of 2λ (0.25 EU/mL) to $\frac{1}{2}\lambda$ (0.0626 EU/mL), which confirms the manufacturer's label claim sensitivity of 0.125 EU/mL. Once confirmed, the label claim sensitivity of 0.125 EU/mL, *not* the determined sensitivity of 0.088 EU/mL, is used for all gel-clot calculations going forward.

Lysates formulated for photometric testing do not have a label claim sensitivity. The sensitivity of the test system, meaning the lowest endotoxin concentration in the maximum recommended standard curve range, is determined by the lysate manufacturer. For any given assay, the test sensitivity (λ) is set by the user, and is equal to the value of the lowest point on the laboratory's referenced standard curve, which might be a subset of the manufacturer's maximum recommended range. To accept a new lot of lysate into the laboratory, the analyst must create a standard curve consisting of at least three points. Most photometric tests suggest a 10-fold dilutions series, though the lysate manufacturer might suggest a twofold series (check the lysate manufacturer's product insert for recommended standard curve parameters).

TABLE 16 Example of a Gel Clot Label Claim Verification Study

Replicate	Endotoxin concentration				Endpoint (EU/mL)	Log endpoint
	2λ (0.25 EU/mL)	λ (0.125 EU/mL)	$\frac{1}{2}\lambda$ (0.0625 EU/mL)	$\frac{1}{4}\lambda$ (0.03125 EU/mL)		
1	+	+	−	−	0.125	−0.093
2	+	−	−	−	0.0625	−1.204
3	+	−	−	−	0.0625	−1.204
4	+	+	−	−	0.125	−0.093

Abbreviation: EU, endotoxin unit.

In order to accept the lot of lysate, the absolute value of the correlation coefficient, or measure of linearity that is calculated from a linear regression analysis of the observed data points, must be greater than or equal to 0.980.

Analyst Qualification

Analyst training is required by the 1987 FDA Guideline, by 21 CFR 211 and by 21 CFR 820 (6–8). Although not specifically required in the harmonized pharmacopeia, the BET analyst qualification exercise, as described in the 1987 FDA Guideline, should be viewed as the culmination of analyst training (6). The essential question in analyst qualification is, "Can each analyst get the same result (label claim for a gel clot test or linearity for a photometric test) as both the lysate manufacturer and the FDA have gotten?" The method for analyst qualification is identical to lysate label claim verification (above).

Endotoxin Standardization

The primary endotoxin standard (RSE) is the endotoxin that lysate manufacturers use to establish label claim (gel clot) or standard curve characteristics (photometric) for each lot of lysate they produce. User laboratories can obtain the consumer version of this standard from USP, but it is expensive and has a relatively short shelf life once reconstituted. Most laboratories opt for using a secondary standard for routine testing called the CSE, obtained from the lysate manufacturer, because it is much less costly and has a longer expiration after reconstitution than the RSE. However, because all of the reagents in the BET are biological in nature, standardization of the potency of the CSE relative to the RSE must be performed for each unique combination of lysate lot/CSE lot in use in the laboratory. In a busy laboratory, this can be quite time consuming and expensive. FDA has historically accepted a certificate of analysis (CoA) obtained from the lysate vendor defining the potency of the CSE in EU/ng for each unique combination of lysate lot/endotoxin lot. It is recommended that the CoA be accepted only after a successful vendor qualification audit (6).

Equipment Qualification

Equipment qualification is a basic component of control in any testing laboratory (3–5,7). For the BET, equipment to be qualified and/or calibrated includes, but may not be limited to, pipettors, heat blocks, water baths, timers, depyrogenation ovens, plate and tube readers, and instrument-specific software. Depyrogenation ovens must have validated time and temperature control specifications for each load pattern the laboratory uses. Heat blocks and water baths used for the incubation of gel clot tests must have current temperature maps to qualify them for use. In addition to heat mapping of the incubating chamber(s), the optics and data transmission for plate and tube readers must be qualified. Software that is used with plate/tube readers for calculation, analysis, and reporting of data must be compliant with 21 CFR Part 11 (10).

Testing of Consumables for Interference with the Test

Many laboratories use plastic consumables in the performance of the BET. These consumables (tubes, pipettes, pipette tips) are received as sterile, but may or may not be free of BET test interference. A label of "pyrogen free" on a consumable is not the same as a lot-specific CoA that reports calculated data obtained from a validated test method. The harmonized BET chapter in the USP, EP, and JP requires that these consumable plastics be tested before use for test interference: essentially leachable inhibitory substances and contaminating surface endotoxin (3–5).

Depyrogenated borosilicate glass is the "gold standard" for the BET. The use of disposable plastic is allowed, but there are cautions. Polystyrene has been shown to be the most benign of the plastics with regard to BET test interference (39,40). Polyproplyene plastic can interfere with the performance of the test, and should be avoided for sample collection and preparation (39,40). An exception to the polypropylene rule is the use of disposable pipette tips for mechanical pipettors. These tips likely do not cause interference because of the short sample exposure time during testing. They should, however, be tested as any other plastic consumable and released prior to use.

There is no published method for the determination of BET interference in plastic consumables. The industry practice, however, is to utilize the same procedure described for the BET testing of medical devices in the United States Pharmacopeia (37). In this method, the product contact surfaces of the test items are exposed to LRW that has been preheated to 37°C. Items are allowed to sit or recirculate (for the examination of fluid pathways) for one hour at controlled room temperature. The soaking water (sometimes called rinse or eluate) is assayed for BET test interference exactly the same way that drug product or a dilution of drug product is tested for interference (below). Demonstration of the lack of test interference (either inhibition or the presence of endogenous endotoxin in the sample) will release the lot of consumables for use in the laboratory.

Depyrogenation

There are two parts to a successful depyrogenation validation study. The first is the physical identification of "cold spots" in the empty chamber and in each load pattern. The second is the demonstration that the chosen time and temperature combination will eliminate endotoxin that is placed in an appropriate pattern to cover all parts of the chamber in a test unit as well as at the cold spots. The rules for depyrogenation are set out in the USP in Chapter $< 1211 >$, "Sterilization and Sterility Assurance of Compendial Articles" (35). Recognizing that endotoxin adsorbs to glass and other surfaces (39,41), the depyrogenation study begins with the demonstration of the recovery of at least 1000 EUs from the surface to be processed. Endotoxin adsorption to surfaces will vary depending on the endotoxin formulation, the endotoxin concentration, the method of fixing endotoxin to the surface, and the recovery method (15,42–44). Aside from the requirement to recover at least 1000 EU/article, there are no rules governing initial concentration, fixing of endotoxin to the surface of the test article, or methods for recovery of endotoxin from the test article, so the laboratory must be able to demonstrate during validation that their spike and recovery methods are valid. A successful depyrogenation requires the demonstration of at least a three-log reduction in endotoxin from the recoverable levels. Log reduction is calculated as follows:

$$\text{Log reduction} = \log_{10} \text{ recoverable endotoxin} - \log_{10} \text{ residual endotoxin}$$
$$\text{(preprocessing)} \qquad \text{(postproccessing)}$$

Example: If testing demonstrates that recoverable endotoxin $= 5000\,\text{EU/unit}$ and residual endotoxin in each test unit is $< 0.03125\,\text{EU/unit}$, the log reduction would be:

- Log reduction $> \log_{10} 5000\,\text{EU} - \log_{10} 0.03125\,\text{EU}$
- Log reduction $> 5 - (-1.5)$

- Log reduction > 6.5
- *Note*: Log reduction > 6.5 because the residual endotoxin is < 0.03125 EU/unit.

Segment 3: Validation

As with the initial QC elements, validation is a requirement of all compendia, lysate manufacturer's product inserts, and the 1987 FDA Guideline, and is therefore a CCP in the preparation for routine use of the BET as a release test or routine monitoring tool. A complete validation study is expected for *any* sample under test, not just for the release of finished drug product.

Validation is the demonstration that the sample under test or a dilution of that sample does not interfere (i.e., neither inhibits nor enhances) with the results of the BET assay. The literature cites many instances of test interference (45,46). Dilution of the product in LRW is the easiest and most convenient way to overcome interference. It makes sense, however, that there be a limit to the allowable dilution so that the limit of detection in the test method is not exceeded. That dilution limit is known as the maximum valid dilution (MVD), and is calculated using the formula:

$$MVD = \frac{(\text{endotoxin limit})(\text{concentration of the product})}{\lambda}$$

where the endotoxin limit $= K/M$, the concentration of the product is equal to the concentration of the active ingredient for those products administered on a weight/kg basis, and equal to 1 for those products administered on a volume/kg basis, $\lambda =$ the test sensitivity, meaning the confirmed label claim sensitivity for gel clot tests, or the lowest point on the referenced standard curve for photometric tests.

In the MVD equation, the endotoxin limit is a constant. As the product concentration increases, so does the MVD. As the test sensitivity increases (i.e., λ gets lower), the MVD increases. The MVD is a dilution factor.

There are two very important system test parameters that need to be met for the BET assay to run optimally (47). The first is pH. It must be demonstrated that the pH of the mixture of sample (or sample dilution) and lysate falls within the optimum range that is specified by the lysate manufacturer. Because the lysate is processed from horseshoe crab blood, it is naturally buffered to some extent, but the final buffering capacity of the reagent depends on the individual lysate manufacturer's product formulation. If the pH of the mixture of lysate and sample falls outside the range, the product may be adjusted using NaOH, HCl, or tris buffers shown to be free of detectable endotoxin, or the sample may be diluted in LRW to reduce the effects of product concentration on pH. The second important test parameter is divalent cations. Divalent cations are important to the lysate reaction, and are added to the lysate during reagent formulation. Those drug products that are chelate (e.g., heparin, citrate or drugs containing EDTA) will lower the divalent ion concentration available for the reaction and may result in an inhibitory response. Adding cations back to the reaction or diluting the product in LRW to reduce the chelating capacity of the test sample are remedies for this interference problem.

Validation requires that the drug product, or dilution of drug product, not exceed the calculated MVD be "spiked" with endotoxin, and that the endotoxin be quantitatively recovered. For gel clot two parallel series of endotoxin dilutions are compared. One series uses LRW as the diluent and acts as the control series. The second series uses drug product diluted to the proposed final test concentration, as the diluent for endotoxin. The geometric mean calculation for the two separate endotoxin dilution series (endotoxin diluted in LRW and endotoxin diluted in product or proposed test concentration of product) must both confirm $\lambda \pm 1$ twofold dilution. For photometric tests, drug product or a dilution of drug product not to exceed the calculated MVD must be spiked at a level equal to the midpoint of the standard curve, and the recovery of the endotoxin spike must be within the range of 50% to 200% of the nominal value (see section "Segment 5: Data Analysis and Interpretation"). Regardless of method, recovery conditions must be met for three lots of drug product. If the test method changes, for example from gel clot to kinetic chromogenic, a new validation must be run on three lots of product. The reason for running a new validation is that the interference profiles of many drug products will change depending on the test method (46).

Segment 4: Routine Testing
Once all of the prerequisites described above in segments 1–3 have been met, the laboratory is ready to test material for release.

System Suitability Control
System suitability control testing is an essential component of a routine BET testing scheme. Properly performed and interpreted system suitability controls help to assure that individual test results are valid. The consequence of inappropriate results on the system suitability is the invalidation of *all* tests that reference those controls. System suitability controls include:

- *Negative control:* The negative control, which is the testing of LRW, assures that the system components (reagents, tubes, technique) do not contribute endotoxin contamination to the test. A valid test requires that the negative control in a gel clot test does not gel and in a photometric test, it does not react.
- *Positive product control (PPC):* A PPC is required for each sample under test. The PPC for a gel clot test is the sample diluted to the test concentration and "spiked" with endotoxin to a level of 2λ. A valid gel clot PPC requires that all tubes containing spiked product gel. For photometric testing, the PPC is the sample diluted to the test concentration "spiked" with endotoxin at a level equal to the midpoint of the standard curve. A valid photometric PPC requires that endotoxin be recovered within the range of 50% to 200% of the nominal spike value.
- *Standard series:* The 1987 FDA Guideline requires that a standard series (2λ, λ, $\frac{1}{2}\lambda$, and $\frac{1}{4}\lambda$) be run at least once a day for each combination of lysate lot/endotoxin lot used in the day's testing. That requirement was dropped in the current harmonized compendial chapters for the limits test. In the harmonized method, a 2λ endotoxin/LRW control is required for each group of limits test

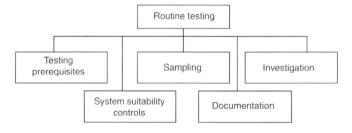

FIGURE 14 Laboratory testing.

samples. The harmonized chapter, however, requires that a standard series be run concurrently with each gel clot assay performed. As in the label claim verification assay, the geometric mean of the standard series must confirm $\lambda \pm 1$ twofold dilution. The standard series for a photometric test is the standard curve. The current harmonized photometric method requires that a standard curve be run for every plate or set of tubes containing test samples. A valid standard curve requires at least three points, and the absolute value of the correlation coefficient, which is a measure of linearity determined from linear regression analysis of those points, must be ≥ 0.980 (3–6).

Sampling

Sampling is not addressed in the harmonized compendia chapters. The only reference to sampling for the BET is found in the 1987 Guideline, which, for drug products, requires that at least three samples be taken to represent the beginning, middle, and end of the filling run. Samples may be pooled for testing or may be tested individually. For medical devices, suggested sampling is based on the lot size (6).

Documentation

Documentation is important for any laboratory test, including the BET. Not only is it good practice to document the specific reagents and materials used to generate any one test result, but these data are important to the investigation of any OOS result or tracking/trending of invalid test results. Depending on the software, much of the following data will be entered into the computer prior to running a photometric test. For gel clot, the data should be kept on controlled laboratory test sheets or laboratory notebooks. Minimally, records should be kept to track the following:

- Reagents used for a particular test, including lot numbers, reconstitution dates, and expiration dates for the lysate, the endotoxin, the LRW, and any other reagents (e.g., buffers, dispersing agents) that might be used in the performance of the test
- Tag numbers for equipment
- Temperature in the incubating device at the beginning and the end of the gel clot test
- Time in/time out for gel clot testing
- Sample identification and lot number for the material under test
- The endotoxin limit, MVD, and test dilution for the sample under test
- Number of samples and whether they are pooled or tested individually
- All raw data results of system suitability testing
- A calculation of the amount of endotoxin measured in the test sample (see section "Segment 5: Data Analysis and Interpretation")
- A final declaration of the status of the test once data are reviewed and compared to product specifications. The declaration should be a choice among the following: meets specification; does not meet specification; invalid; needs investigation.

Investigation

The laboratory must have a provision for investigation in the event of a test failure. An OOS on the BET is a de facto sample failure unless the result can be unequivocally shown to be due to a documented laboratory error. The investigation may be divided into two parts. The first is a review of all of the laboratory data including system suitability, calibration/qualification status, and/or maintenance record of the equipment used in the performance of the test, the history of the lots of reagents used, and analyst interview. The purpose of this part of the investigation is to determine if the OOS was due to a testing error. Some examples of invalid tests:

- Nonconforming system suitability results
- A depyrogenation cycle for the reaction tubes (gel clot) or sample preparation materials (tubes, spatulas, etc.) that did not meet time/temperature specifications
- The observation, at the end of the test period, that the volume of liquid in the well or tube is inappropriate (i.e., visibly too high or too low)
- Analyst testing history—Has this analyst had more than his/her share of OOS and/or invalid test results? Is retraining necessary?

The second part of the investigation is a full inquiry into the manufacture of the drug product. Referencing back to the process HACCP and the corresponding CCPs with regard to the endotoxin hazard provides the basis for this part of the investigation. This portion of the investigation should include (but should not necessarily be limited to):

1. Results of CCP raw material and in-process testing relative to established endotoxin limits
2. Results of WFI testing
3. Results of CIP/SIP
4. Examination of the depyrogenation processes for sampling and manufacturing equipment
5. Examination of the any product stream depyrogenation steps
6. Examination of environmental monitoring results for the presence of gram-negative bacteria in the manufacturing area
7. Examination of batch records to identify other hazard excursions or processing interventions that might be related to the endotoxin OOS
8. Trending of data over the last three, six, and 12 months relative to:

   - Sample type—Has this sample type had relatively more OOS/invalid test results than others? Has there been a process change that could warrant additional validation testing? Has endotoxin in this sample type been trending upward (or downward), even if it has not exceeded established action limits?
   - Manufacturing personnel—Have the same personnel been involved in previous BET OOS results? If so, should they be retrained?
   - Manufacturing equipment—Examine the maintenance record of laboratory and manufacturing equipment. Might there be a problem with equipment that could contribute to the problem?

Segment 5: Data Analysis and Interpretation

End-Product Testing
The focus of the testing laboratory is to keep control over the test conditions and methods to assure that results are accurate, precise, and consistent. Accuracy and precision are measures of experimental error. Consistency is inter/intra-analyst or inter/intralaboratory reproducibility. Misinterpretation or miscalculation of data can lead to false results—both false positive and false negative. To that end, the data analysis and interpretation are CCPs.

Precision is a measure of the reproducibility of measurements with a data set. In a gel clot, confirmation of label claim limits imprecision because a valid test requires that the geometric mean of the standard series confirm the label claim ± 1 twofold dilution. To analytical chemists, a ± 1 twofold dilution is a huge error—it allows for a maximum error of 100%! But remember, this is a biological assay, not an analytical assay. In photometric tests, the coefficient of variation for replicate sample aliquots is the measure of precision.

Accuracy is a measure of how close a data point or calculated value is to a reference value—a theoretical value, a known value, or a hypothetical value. Label claim in gel clot requires that the analyst confirm an external value—the label claim that was initially assigned by the lysate manufacturer, confirmed by CBER, and ultimately confirmed by the testing laboratory. In kinetics, there is no requirement to "match" any standard curve parameter to a value supplied by the manufacturer. Is this a problem? Consider the following kinetic test. The thin solid line in Figure 15 represents a linear kinetic standard curve. The dashed line represents the onset time and interpolated value of an unknown (x). If we acknowledge that the sample onset time is independent of the standard curve to which it is compared, we can see that the same sample onset time, when interpolated from another standard curve (thick line), will give us a very different result (y), in this case an underestimation of endotoxin content which, depending on the endotoxin limit for the product, may be a false negative result. Likewise, if the sample onset time is interpolated from the thick dotted line, we might get an overestimation of endotoxin in the sample (z), which, depending on the endotoxin limit for the product may be a false positive result.

In this case, the standard curves that resulted in an overestimation ("z") or underestimation ("y") both met the linearity requirement and had the same slope as the first standard curve, but the y-intercept was different. Therefore, the differences among the interpolated values "x," "y," and "z" are not differences in onset times or endotoxin levels, but they are artifacts of uncontrolled standard curves. What could cause a change in the y-intercept? The inappropriate dilution of standards. Weak standards will overestimate endotoxin. Strong standards will underestimate endotoxin.

Two other standard curve parameters that could affect the calculation of endotoxin levels in unknowns are linearity and slope.

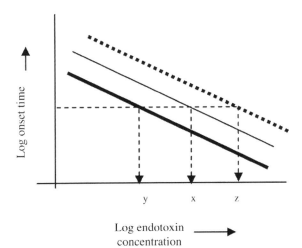

Log onset time

Log endotoxin concentration

FIGURE 15 The effect of y-intercept on endotoxin determination.

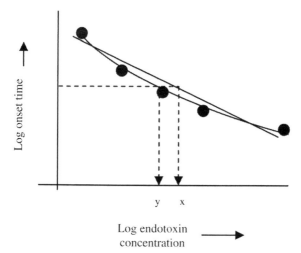

Log endotoxin concentration ⟶

FIGURE 16 The effect of linearity on endotoxin determination.

The standard curves for endotoxin assays are often bowed. This nonlinearity is a function of the nature of the assay, as well as the range of the standard curve (wider range standard curves tend to be less linear). Figure 16 shows two curves: a "bowed" curve that could well be the curve that results from the observed points and a linear curve, the curve that might be determined from the linear regression analysis of the observed points; "x" is the level of endotoxin interpolated from the standard curve; "y" is the endotoxin level that would be expected relative to the observed points. The greater the bow, the greater the inaccuracy of the interpolated value (48–50). Nonlinearity can be addressed by (i) limiting the range of the standard curve and/or (ii) using a polynomial regression rather than a linear regression curve analysis tool.[d]

The third parameter in photometric testing than can result in "false" or inaccurate results is slope. Figure 17 shows two standard curves that both meet the linearity requirement and that share the same y-intercept. However, they differ in slope. A number of standard-curve related issues are illustrated in Figure 17.

■ The onset time for sample "a" is greater than the bottom point on the thin line standard curve, meaning that the sample has less than λ endotoxin ($\lambda =$ the bottom point on the standard curve). For example, if the standard curve were 5.0 EU/mL - 0.05 EU/mL (λ), the sample onset time, as interpolated from the thin line standard curve, would be recorded as < 0.05 EU/mL. However, if the same onset time were used to interpolate and calculate an endotoxin result from the thick standard curve, there would be detectable endotoxin in the sample. If this were a water sample, the result could be pass or fail depending on a firm's WFI limit the referenced standard curve.

■ Likewise, the onset time for sample "b" indicates that again, the endotoxin content could be significantly different depending on the referenced standard curve.

---

[d] The use of polynomial regression is approved by the FDA on a lysate manufacturer-by-manufacturer basis. Contact your lysate manufacturer for details.

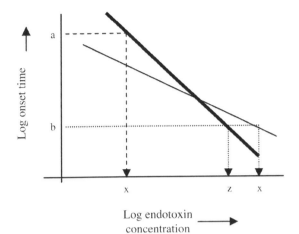

Log onset time

a

b

x   z   x

Log endotoxin
concentration

FIGURE 17 The effect of slope on
endotoxin determination.

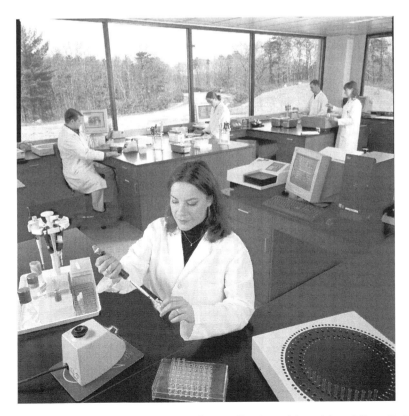

FIGURE 18 LAL Testing Laboratory. *Source*: Courtesy of Associates of Cape Cod, Inc.

Accuracy in endotoxin determination in the photometric test is a function of the accuracy of the standard curve. Laboratories must be cognizant of the effects that standard curves parameters (y-intercept, slope, linearity) can have on test results, and must work toward limiting the allowable divergence in these parameters from day to day between analysts and between instruments.

Tracking and Trending

Tracking and trending of OOS results and the accompanying investigation reports and CAPAs is routine in the parenteral industry. However, laboratories often forget to track/trend laboratory errors and take the time to deduce the reasons for invalid test results. For example, Table 17 is a listing of all of the invalid kinetic testing results from a fictional laboratory.

Looking at the data chronologically, one can see that there were many problems in 2003, but trends, patterns, but the possible or probable root causes are not obvious. If the table were sorted first by problem and then by analyst, a very different pattern emerges (Table 18).

A number of patterns are now obvious. Clearly, attention to these trends and the immediate implementation of appropriate preventive actions will reduce the risk of invalid and/or "false" results in the future.

- All of the "hot wells" (presumed random endotoxin contamination in microwell plates) were attributed to CC. Is this really a "hot well" problem, or is it an analyst problem?
- BA was responsible for 5/7 or 71% of the invalid spike recoveries. Does he need retraining?

TABLE 17 Invalid Test Results for 2003

Date	Problem	Lysate lot	Analyst	Product	Correlation
12/31/2003	Invalid spike	XYZ123	BA	WFI port 2	0.991
1/14/2003	OOS	XYZ123	KS	Holding tank	0.998
2/11/2003	Void curve	XYZ123	BA	N/A	0.979
2/13/2003	Hot well	XYZ123	CC	NSA	0.999
2/21/2003	Invalid spike	XYZ123	BA	Lipid emulsion	0.995
3/16/2003	OOS	XYZ123	CC	Ampicillin	0.999
3/31/2003	Invalid spike	XYZ123	BA	NSA	0.986
4/4/2003	Negative cont	XYZ123	MG	NaCl	0.996
4/30/2003	Hot well	XYZ123	CC	WFI port 2	0.999
5/8/2003	OOS	XYZ123	BA	Holding tank	0.997
5/28/2003	Invalid spike	ABC234	BA	Ringer's	0.993
6/7/2003	Invalid spike	ABC234	MG	Lipid emulsion	0.999
6/13/2003	Hot well	ABC234	CC	Recrystallized	0.986
7/4/2003	OOS	ABC234	MG	Holding tank	0.999
8/29/2003	Missed well	ABC234	KS	Ampicillin	0.994
9/2/2003	Void curve	ABC234	BA	Ringer's	0.976
9/12/2003	Negative cont	ABC234	KS	WFI port 2	0.998
10/6/2003	Hot well	ABC234	CC	NaCl	0.999
10/30/2003	Invalid spike	ABC234	BA	Holding tank	0.991
11/4/2003	Invalid spike	ABC234	CC	Lipid emulsion	1.000
11/24/2003	OOS	ABC234	KS	Holding tank	0.998
12/14/2003	Negative cont	ABC234	MG	NSA	0.997
12/30/2003	Void curve	ABC234	BA	NaCl	0.975

Abbreviations: OOS, out of specification; WFI, water for injection.

TABLE 18 Invalid Test Results for 2003 Sorted by Problem and Analyst

Date	Problem	Lysate lot	Analyst	Product	Correlation
2/13/2003	Hot well	XYZ123	CC	NSA	0.999
4/30/2003	Hot well	XYZ123	CC	WFI port 2	0.999
6/13/2003	Hot well	ABC234	CC	Recrystallized	0.986
10/6/2003	Hot well	ABC234	CC	NaCl	0.999
12/31/2003	Invalid spike	XYZ123	BA	WFI port 2	0.991
2/21/2003	Invalid spike	XYZ123	BA	Lipid emulsion	0.995
3/31/2003	Invalid spike	XYZ123	BA	NSA	0.986
5/28/2003	Invalid spike	ABC234	BA	Ringer's	0.993
10/30/2003	Invalid spike	ABC234	BA	Holding tank	0.991
11/4/2003	Invalid spike	ABC234	CC	Lipid emulsion	1.000
6/7/2003	Invalid spike	ABC234	MG	Lipid emulsion	0.999
8/29/2003	Missed well	ABC234	KS	Ampicillin	0.994
9/12/2003	Negative cont	ABC234	KS	WFI port 2	0.998
4/4/2003	Negative cont	XYZ123	MG	NaCl	0.996
12/14/2003	Negative cont	ABC234	MG	NSA	0.997
5/8/2003	OOS	XYZ123	BA	Holding tank	0.997
3/16/2003	OOS	XYZ123	CC	Ampicillin	0.999
1/14/2003	OOS	XYZ123	KS	Holding tank	0.998
11/24/2003	OOS	ABC234	KS	Holding tank	0.998
7/4/2003	OOS	ABC234	MG	Holding tank	0.999
2/11/2003	Void curve	XYZ123	BA	N/A	0.979
9/2/2003	Void curve	ABC234	BA	Ringer's	0.976
12/30/2003	Void curve	ABC234	BA	NaCl	0.975

Abbreviations: OOS, out of specification; WFI, water for injection.

- Looking more closely at the invalid spike recoveries, 3/7 or roughly 43% of the invalid spike recoveries were with lipid emulsion. These three invalid spikes were obtained by three different analysts. Could this trend indicate a problem with interference in the assay? Was there a change in a process step or raw material that could correlate with the issues with lipid emulsion spike recovery?
- MG was responsible for 66% of the negative control problems. Does he need retraining?
- Sixty percent of the OOS results were on WFI holding tank samples. Is there a larger problem with the holding tank? Did these OOS results occur after shutdowns? After cleanings? What about products made on those days? What did the loop samples look like on those days? Is there a problem with access to the holding tank port that could cause a sampling error and result in endotoxin contamination?
- BA as responsible for 100% of the voided curves, which were the result of non-linearity. Remember, BA was also responsible for 71% of the invalid spike recoveries (above). Do we have a problem with BA?

SUMMARY

This chapter has demonstrated the application of HACCP as one method of risk analysis to apply the bacterial endotoxin test as a tool for process control. Once our assumptions and "knowns" were clearly delineated, HACCP helped to objectively identify and differentiate CCPs in the process. The exercise forced us to think carefully about every step in the manufacturing process. Perhaps not unexpectedly, HACCP indicated that the laboratory testing of the product is just as critical, arguably more critical, than the processing itself in determining the fate of a drug product.

The identification of these points through HACCP is an invaluable asset in the analysis of product and process throughout the product life cycle. In development, the analysis will help to identify potential processing inconsistencies. During technology transfer and validation, the analysis helps to identify a minimal but valuable number of significant focus points. For routine testing, HACCP forced us to think carefully and assign scientifically sound and attainable endotoxin limits to CCPs.

ABBREVIATIONS AND ACRONYMS

API	Active pharmaceutical ingredient
BET	Bacterial endotoxins test
CAPA	Corrective action/preventive action
CBER	Center for biologics evaluation and research
CCP	Critical control point
CFR	Code of federal regulations
CIP	Clean in place
cGMP	Current good manufacturing practices
CoA	Certificate of analysis
CP	Control point
EP	European Pharmacopeia
EU	Endotoxin unit
GMP	Good Manufacturing Practices
HACCP	Hazard and critical control point analysis
HVAC	Heating, ventilation and air conditioning
IM	Intramuscular
IV	Intravenous
IVD	In vitro diagnostic
ISO	International Organization for Standardization
JP	Japanese Pharmacopeia
LAL	Limulus amebocyte lysate
LOQ	Limit of quantitation
LPS	Lipopolysaccharide
LRW	LAL reagent water
LVP	Large volume parenteral
MVD	Maximum valid dilution
OOS	Out of specification
OOT	Out of trend
PDA	Parenteral drug association
PPC	Positive product control
QA	Quality assurance
QC	Quality control
QSR	Quality system regulation
RODAC	Replicate organism detection and counting (plates)
SIP	Sterilize in place
SVP	Small volume parenteral
USP	U.S. Pharmacopeia
WFI	Water for injection

GLOSSARY

Bracket — A term used to describe the series of endotoxin dilutions used in gel clot testing. Bracketing means preparing endotoxin dilutions equal to 2λ, λ, $\frac{1}{2}\lambda$ and $\frac{1}{4}\lambda$ where λ is equal to the label claim sensitivity of a gel clot reagent

Correlation coefficient — A measure of linearity that is calculated from the linear regression of a set of observed points. A correlation coefficient of $|1.0|$ means that the observed points statistically fall directly on the regression line

Endotoxin — A potent class of pyrogens isolated from the outer cell membrane of gram-negative bacteria

Endotoxin limit — The maximum allowable level of endotoxin for a product with a specific formula and an identified maximum dose

Endpoint — For the gel clot test, the endpoint is the last positive that is followed by a negative in a series of endotoxin dilutions

Failure mode — A design failure in which a system, subsystem, process or part fails to meet its intended purpose or function (30)

Good manufacturing practice — Defined in 21 CFR 211, good manufacturing practices (GMP) describe accepted and expected principles and practices for the manufacture of parenteral drug products

Hazard — Any condition that results in an adverse consequence that is detrimental to the product, the end user, or the manufacturer

Lambda (λ) — The BET test sensitivity defined as the confirmed label claim sensitivity for gel clot and the lowest point on the referenced standard curve for photometric methods

Limulus amebocyte lysate (LAL) reagent water (LRW) — LAL reagent water is water containing no detectable endotoxin in the LAL test system. LRW is used for the BET negative control

Lipopolysaccharide — The chemical description of purified endotoxin

Pyrogen — A fever-causing substance

Quality system — Defined in 21 CFR 820, the Quality System is the current GMP for medical devices

Risk — The estimation of the possible occurrence of an identified hazard or hazardous condition

Risk analysis — Examination of a combination of empirical data, scientifically based assumptions, manufacturing experience and compliance requirements to determine risk

Risk control — Proactive measures taken to restrict the possibility of risk in a manufacturing operation

Risk management — The process of understanding, anticipating, and minimizing the potential impact of a product failure or hazard to the product, the end user, or the manufacturer

Spike — The addition of a known amount of endotoxin to a test article

Ultrafiltration — A filtration process whereby molecules are excluded based on their molecular weight. Ultrafilters are rated on the basis of molecular weight exclusion limits, and their effectiveness as depyrogenating filters is due to their action as size-discriminating screens (12)

REFERENCES

1. United States Food and Drug Administration. Pharmaceutical cGMPs for the 21st Century: A Risk Based Approach 2002 at http://www.fda.gov/od/guidance/gmp.html.
2. United States Food and Drug Administration. Pharmaceutical cGMPs for the 21st Century: A Risk Based Approach: Second Progress Report and Implementation Plan 2002 at http://www.fda.gov.cdergmp21stcenturysummary.htm.
3. United States Pharmacopeia. "Bacterial Endotoxin Test" 2004a; 27:85.
4. European Pharmacopeia. Chapter 2,6,14, "Bacterial Endotoxins", 2002.
5. Japanese Pharmacopeia. "Bacterial Endotoxins Test". Chap. 6, 2001.
6. United States Food and Drug Administration. Guideline on Validation of the Limulus Amebocyte Lysate Test as an Enroduct Endotoxin Test for Human and Animal Parenteral Drugs, Biological Products, and Medical Devices, 1987 at http://www.fda.gov/cder/guidance/old005fn.pdf.
7. Code of Federal Regulations. Current Good Manufacturing Practices for Finished Pharmaceuticals.Title 21, Part 211. 2003a.
8. Code of Federal Regulations. Electronic Records; Electronic Signatures. Title 21, Part 11. 2003b.
9. Code of Federal Regulations. Good Laboratory Practice for Nonclinical Laboratory Studies Title 21, Part 58. 2003c.
10. Code of Federal Regulations. Quality System Regulation Title 21, Part 820. 2003d.
11. Williams KL. Endotoxins: Pyrogens, LAL Testing and Depyrogenation. 2nd ed. New York: Marcel Dekker, 2001.
12. Pearson FC. Pyrogens: Endotoxins, LAL Testing and Depyrogenation. New York: Marcel Dekker inc, 1985:32.
13. Parenteral Drug Association. Technical Monograph #7. Depyrogenation, 1985.
14. Weary M, Pearson F III. A manufacturer's guide to depyrogenation. BioPharm 1988; 1[4]:22–29.
15. LAL Users' Group. Preparation and use of endotoxin indicators for depyrogenation process studies. J Parent Sci Tech 1989; 43(3):109–112.
16. Dabbah R, Ferry E Jr, Gunther DA, et al. Pyrogenicity of *E. coli* 055:B5 endotoxin by the USP rabbit test–a HIMA collaborative study. J Parenter Drug Assoc 1980; 34(3):212–216.
17. Hochstein HD, Fitzgerald EA, McMahon FG, Vargas R. Properties of US Standard endotoxin (E) in human male volunteers. J Endotoxin Res 1994; 1:52–56.
18. Weary M. Understanding and setting endotoxin limits. J Parent Sci Tech 1990; 44(1):16.
19. United States Pharmacopeia 29, < 85 > . Bacterial Endotoxin Test 2006.
20. McCullough KZ. Process control: in process and raw material testing using LAL. Pharma Technol 1988:40.
21. United States Food and Drug Administration. Guide to Inspection of Quality Systems, 1999 at http://www.fda.gov/ora/inspect_ref/igs/qsit/qsitguide.htm.
22. United States Food and Drug Administration. Quality System Manual, 1997b at http://www.fda.gov/cdrh/qsr.
23. United States Food-Drug Administration. Guidance for Industry Sterile Drugs Produced by Aseptic Processing Current Good Manufacturing Practice 2004.
24. United States Food and Drug Administration. Hazard Analysis and Critical Control Point Principles and Application Guidelines, 1997a at http://www.cfsan.fda.gov/~comm/nacmcfp.html.

25. European Parliament and the Council of the European Union. 1998. Directive 98/79/EC of the European Parliament and of the Council of 27 October 1998 on in vitro diagnostic medical devices.
26. International Organization for Standardization (ISO). International Standard 14971, "Application of the concepts of risk management to medical devices", 2000.
27. European Diagnostic Manufacturer's Organization. Risk Analysis of In Vitro Diagnostic Medical Devices, 1998.
28. American Society for Quality. The Certified Quality Auditor's HACCP Handbook. Milwaukee, Wisconsin: ASQ Quality Press, 2002.
29. Corlett DA. HACCP User's Manual. Gaithersburg, Maryland: Aspen Publishers Inc, 1998.
30. Stamatis DH. Failure Mode and Effect Analysis: FMEA from theory to execution. 2nd ed. Milwaukee, Wisconsin: ASQ Quality Press, 2003.
31. NACMCF. 1992. Hazard analysis and Critical Control Point Principles and Application Guidelines. National Advisory Committee on Microbiological Criteria for Foods.
32. McCullough KZ, John TS. Microbial attributes of active pharmaceutical ingredients. In: Ira Berry, Daniel Harpaz, ed. Validating Active Pharmaceutical Ingredients. Denver, Colorado: IHS Health Group, 2001.
33. Sweadner KJ, Forte M, Nelson LL. Filtration removal of endotoxin (pyrogens) in solution in different states of aggregation. Appl Env Microbiol 1992; 34:382–395.
34. Abramson D, Butler LD, Chrai S. Depyrogenation of a parenteral solution by ultrafiltration. J Parent Sci Tech 1981; 35:3–7.
35. United States Pharmacopeia "Sterilization and sterility assurance of compendial articles" 2004c; 27:1211.
36. United States Food and Drug Administration. Guidance for Industry: Investigating Out of Specification (OOS) Test Results for Pharmaceutical Production 1998 at http://www.fda.gov/cder/guidance1212dft.pdf.
37. United States Pharmacopeia. "Transfusion and Infusion Assemblies and Similar Medical Devices" 2004b; 27:161.
38. Levin J, Bang F. Clottable protein in Limulus: Its localization and kinetics of its coagulation by endotoxin. Thromb Diath Haemorrh 1968; 19:186–197.
39. Roslansky PF, Dawson ME, Novitsky TG. Plastics, endotoxins, and the limulus amebocyte lysate test. J Parent Sci Tech 1991; 45:83–87.
40. Novitsky TJ. 1988. The Problems with Plastics In, LAL update Vol 6, No. 3.
41. Roslansky PF, Dawson ME, Novitsky TJ. Problems with plastic test tubes. J Cell Biol 1990; 3:308.
42. Novitsky TJ, Schmidengenback J, Remillard JF. Factors affecting recovery of endotoxin adsorbed to container surfaces. J Parent Sci Tech 1986; 40(6).
43. Jensch UE, Gail L, Klaoehn M. Fixing and removing of bacterial endotoxin from glass surfaces for validation of dry heat sterilization. In: Detection of Bacterial Endotoxins with the Limulus Amebocyte Lysate Test. New York: Alan R Liss, 1987.
44. Ludwig JD, Avis KV. Validation of a heating cell for precisely controlled studies on the thermal destruction of endotoxin in glass. J Parent Sci Tech 1986; 42(1).
45. Twohy CW, Duran AP, Munson TE. Endotoxin contamination of parenteral drugs and radiopharmaceuticals as determined by the limulus amebocyte lysate method. J Parent Sci Tech 1984; 38:190–201.
46. McCullough KZ, Cynthia W. Variability in the LAL test: comparison of three kinetic methods for the testing of pharmaceutical products. J Parent Sci Tech 1992; 44:69–72.
47. Cooper JF. Resolving LAL test interferences. J Parent Sci Tech 1990; 44(1):13–15.

48. Associates of Cape Cod. LAL Update 1998; 16(4). http://www.acciusa.com/pdf/updat1298.pdf.

49. Charles River Endosafe. LAL Times, 2000. http://www.criver.com/endosafe/techdocsendo_pdf/LAL_Times_Sept2000.pdf.

50. Cambrex Biosciences. Win CL Software, 2004. http://www.cambrex.com/Content/Documents/Bioscience/Automated%LAL%20Software.pdf.

51. European Commission. EC Guide to Good Manufacturing Practice. Revision to Annex 1. Manufacture of Sterile Medicinal Products, 2003.

52. United States of America, Plantiff vs Barr Laboratories, Inc et al, Dependants. Civic Action 92-1744.

9 Fault Tree Analysis of the United States Pharmacopeia Sterility Test

Karen Zink McCullough and Audra Zakzeski

Fault Tree Analysis of the United States Pharmacopeia Sterility Test

Karen Zink McCullough
Whitehouse Station, New Jersey, U.S.A.

Audra Zakzeski
Carson City, Nevada, U.S.A.

INTRODUCTION

A "necessary evil" is something that one does not like to do, or perhaps does not understand the need to do, but which one realizes must be done. Sterility testing falls into this category. It must be done because the Code of Federal Regulations (CFR) requires that a sterility test be performed on each lot of product labeled "sterile" (21 CFR 211.167(a); 21 CFR 610.12). Unfortunately, given the statistical limitations of the current test method, the result of a sterility test really gives little, if any, indication about the sterility of a batch (Appendix 1) (1,2).

> Statistical evaluations indicate ... if a 10,000-unit lot with a 0.1 percent contamination level was sterility tested using 20 units, there is a 98 percent chance that the batch would pass the test (1).

Given these statistics, it is reasonable to assert that sterility is assured through careful process validation and control, not through end product testing.

A positive result on a sterility test presents the manufacturer with a quandary—was the test contaminated by the analyst during test execution or was it randomly contaminated at any number of critical steps during manufacture or is there a systemic problem that could have caused the failure? A failed sterility test is considered by Food and Drug Administration and by United States Pharmacopeia (USP) to be "guilty until proven innocent" and the assumption is that the contamination took place at some point during manufacture unless and until it can be proven conclusively that the failure was caused by a deficiency in the laboratory (1,3,4). 21 CFR 211.165(f) states, "Drug products failing to meet established standards or specifications and any other relevant quality control criteria shall be rejected." Thus, any failed sterility test carries significant financial and compliance implications for the drug manufacturer.

As sterility is a quality attribute of parenteral products, a failure is, by definition, out-of-specification (OOS) result and is subject to extensive investigation, regardless of the lot's ultimate disposition (5,6). The investigation must be unbiased, scientifically sound, and timely. It must not only look for the cause of the failed test in question, but also should use the failure as a starting point for looking for adverse trends or patterns in laboratory test results, environmental monitoring data, manufacturing batch records, facility-monitoring data such as temperature and humidity, and validated systems such as water for injection (WFI). The investigation must be supported by the collection of "objective evidence," and should include any corrective action or preventive action (CAPA) that becomes evident as a result of the analysis (1,3,4,6–8).

Practically speaking, an investigation into a failed sterility test is more of a preventive exercise than a corrective one. It is extraordinarily difficult to justify the invalidation of a failed sterility test. If your only purpose in performing an investigation into laboratory testing is to invalidate a failed test, you will likely be disappointed in your efforts. However, the investigation process can be a most productive one if it leads to a better understanding of both the manufacturing and the sterility test processes and identifies activities, situations, equipment, or processes that can be improved upon in order to prevent another OOS from happening.

RISK

In the best of all worlds, a manufacturer will perform a risk analysis during developments scale up and transfer of the product for routine manufacture. This risk analysis is a cross-functional effort with representation from development, manufacturing/operations, quality, engineering, and facilities to identify critical processing points relative to identified product hazards or failure modes. For the purposes of this chapter, our failure is a nonsterile product. The risk analysis can be performed using any number of published models including hazard analysis and critical control point (HACCP), failure modes and effects analysis (FMEA), or fault tree analysis (FTA) to identify process critical control points or faults that could be root causes of a an identified failure (9–12). The utility of performing a prospective risk analysis is clear.

- Critical points in the manufacture and testing of the product relative to any identified hazard or failure mode can be objectively identified for the purposes of process validation, process control/monitoring, and test method development.
- Limits for both validation and routine monitoring can be set for all identified critical points.
- Validation and routine documentation requirements for monitoring of critical points can be identified.
- Provisions for trending of data from critical monitoring points can be described.
- The prospective risk analysis provides a consensus-driven, consistent, unbiased, and scientifically based roadmap for an investigation in the event of a test failure.

Risk analysis does not only applied to manufacturing processes. The microbiology laboratory should perform a risk analysis on critical methods such as sterility testing in order to prospectively identify and proactively correct or control potential problems that could result in an OOS sterility test result.

This chapter takes a critical look at sterility test methodology from the perspective of a failure. We have chosen FTA as our tool, although any risk analysis tool can be adapted for this purpose. Throughout this chapter, we describe the types of objective evidence that might be collected in support of the investigation and CAPAs that might be proposed if the evidence suggests a deficiency. Our examples are only illustrative, as the required or desired objective evidence and CAPAs will vary with the product, the process, the facility, etc. As a cautionary note, we focus here on the laboratory portion of the investigation. As a sterility failure can have more than one identified root cause, a complete investigation contains rigorous analyses of all possible root causes in the lab, manufacturing, and facilities. For those who are unfamiliar with sterility test, Appendix 1 provides a discussion of the basic components of the test procedure and test interpretation. (Appendix 2 provides some insight into the statistical basis and limitations of the current test method as described in USP 29 (4).)

THE STERILITY TEST FAILURE CASE STUDY

Root Cause Determination via Fault Tree Analysis

With the observation of an OOS result, we are obligated by 21 CFR 211.192, legal precedent, FDA, and our own standard operating procedures (SOPs) to determine the root cause(s) of any sterility test failure (1,5,6). Root cause analysis will help us to identify the who, what, where, when, why, and how of a failure and in the process will provide clues for generating CAPAs that will address deficiencies with an eye toward preventing similar failures from happening in the future (13). How do we approach and document our thought process through to the identification of a root cause of the failure?

The investigation is optimally driven by quality assurance (QA). Why QA? Since they neither manufacture nor test the product, they have no "stake" in the outcome of the investigation other than to assure that it is objective, scientific, and timely. Recognizing that there may be more than one root cause for the failure and given the goal to provide an unbiased and scientific analysis of the failure, the investigation team should be cross-functional, and should require participation by affected departments including manufacturing/operations, quality control/testing, engineering, and facilities (6).

We have chosen a method called "fault tree analysis" or FTA for our example. FTA is a "top-down," deductive, qualitative approach to failure analysis (12). The "language" of FTA, as adapted for our purposes, is simple. The sterility failure is the top event. We look to analyze the failure through the identification of increasingly more specific intermediate events that could potentially contribute to the failure. Each intermediate event could have additional contributing input events. The relationship between input and output events is described by a gate. For our example, we will rely on the "OR" gate described in Table 1. In the end, we identify a series of basic events as potential root causes of the failure. This collection of basic events is our unbiased set of possible root cause events that we will use to steer the investigation. The complete graphic representation of possible faults for the identified failure will serve to highlight the interrelationships between departments, procedures, and events when prospectively analyzing a process or retrospectively investigating a failure.

TABLE 1 Symbols Used in Fault Tree Analysis

Symbol	Meaning
□	An intermediate event—an event that occurs because of one or more causes active through logic gates
a⌂	An "OR" gate—the output from this gate occurs if at least one of the inputs occurs
a◯	A "basic event"—identifies a basic initiating fault with no further development (i.e., "end of the line" for that particular branch of our analysis)

The three basic symbols that we are using and their meanings are described below and in Ref. (12):

The Investigation

At a very high level, there are three basic sources of error that could have resulted in a sterility OOS: either there was a problem with the analysis itself (laboratory-related), and/or there was an isolated and potentially identifiable error associated only with the manufacturing of the batch in question (operator or nonprocess-related error), and/or there was a batch-independent chronic problem with a process, procedure, or system (process-related error) (5). Supporting any OOS investigation is the collection and analysis of "objective evidence," which is documentation that will become part of the investigation record and must be used in the justification for excluding or implicating any basic event as a possible root cause of the failure.

Preliminary Analysis

To support the formal investigation, it is prudent to take time to look at the sterility failure in the context of the history of testing, the product tested, any changes to the product or process, and the type of organism that has been identified (Table 2). This initial examination of historic trends is not the complete investigation, but it provides a perspective for the investigation that could provide some clues for specific questions to ask and additional data to gather and analyze in the performance of the remainder of the inquiry?

In the end, the failure could be the result of a combination of laboratory, process, and nonprocess-related errors. In the event of multiple root cause determinations, process and nonprocess-related errors "trump" laboratory errors, and the batch must be rejected.

The Fault Tree

The beginning of the fault tree might look like Figure 1. The top event is the sterility test failure. The three big intermediate categories that could contribute to the failure are laboratory errors, nonprocess-related batch-specific isolated errors, and batch-independent or systemic process-related errors. We will work through the possibility of laboratory error (Fig. 1), but a complete investigation would work through all three error categories.

Laboratory Error

If we consider the laboratory as a potential source of error, we must ask the questions, "What behaviors, conditions, or procedures in the testing laboratory could result in an inadvertent contamination event and nonproduct-related growth in a sterility test?" and "What was different or unique about this particular test and its supporting functions that could have contributed to the OOS?"

We have identified six major categories of possible causes, faults, or clues that could help us to determine if our failure is laboratory-related: (i) test method, (ii) organism identification (ID), (iii) transport of materials used in the performance of the test, (iv) equipment used in the performance of the test, (v) the environment in the sterility test suite, and (vi) the analyst's technique in the performance of the test. We consistently use the "or" gate symbol in our graphic, because there may ultimately be more than one intermediate event or root cause (Fig. 2).

TABLE 2 Preliminary Analysis: Looking at Historical Trends

Trends in ...	... could indicate
Sterility OOS by product type (e.g., lyophilized, terminally sterilized, aseptically manufactured)	Process error (terminal sterilization cycle needs revalidation, transfer of filled vials from filling machine to the lyophilizer is not monitored)
Sterility OOS by a specific product	Process error (manufacturing process)
Sterility OOS by analyst	Laboratory error (difficulty in test method)
Sterility OOS by season	Process error (facility issue)
	Nonprocess error (e.g., seasonally high bioburden in raw materials)
	Laboratory error (poor control of environment)
Sterility OOS correlated with trends or spikes in manufacturing environmental monitoring	Process error (chronic facility control problem)
	Nonprocess error (spikes in EM could indicate acute nonprocess problem involving facilities or people)
Sterility OOS correlated with trends or spikes in testing suite environmental monitoring	Laboratory error (failure to control the testing environment)
Sterility OOS correlated with "people" organisms	Nonprocess error (poor hygiene, poor aseptic technique, poor cleanroom etiquette)
	Process error (poor cleaning regimen)
	Laboratory error (poor aseptic technique on the part of the analyst)
Sterility OOS correlated with "environmental" organisms	Process error (poor cleaning regimen, poor sterilization regimen, poor facility control)
Sterility OOS correlated with time of the day that the test is performed	Laboratory error (could be associated with lack of control of temperature and humidity in the test area; could be associated with fatigue on the part of the analyst)
	Sterility OOS correlated with change in process, raw material supplier
	Process error (poor validation, poor vendor qualification)
Sterility OOS correlated with manufacturing shift	Nonprocess error (potentially personnel-related)

Abbreviations: OOS, out-of-specification; EM, environmental monitoring.

TEST METHOD

A valid sterility test method requires considerable supporting work and documentation (4). We can identify two broad classes of supporting data: test method validation and routine system suitability tests (Fig. 3).

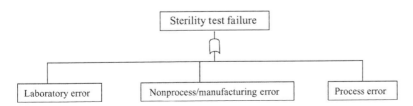

FIGURE 1

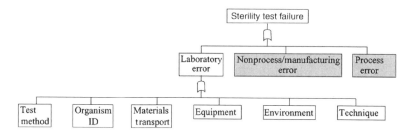

FIGURE 2

Test Method Validation

The validation of the test method answers the question, "Is there any interference in the test system that would prevent the growth of microorganisms?" Quite honestly, the risk in not performing a validation of the sterility test method is a false-negative result (due to undetected test inhibition), not a false-positive (14,15). But, as GMP requires that all test methods be validated, it is an important basic premise of any investigation to demonstrate the validity of a test method. As with any analytical method, the sterility test should not be performed in the absence of a validation study.

Objective evidence:

■ A properly executed and documented validation study must be filed for each product that is subject to sterility testing to assure that the test performs as expected.
■ A check of the testing SOP and an interview with the analyst may reveal that the validated test method was not followed. If this is the case, there is the possibility that an extra step was added or a step was deleted that could have caused an inadvertent contamination event.

Corrective action (or) preventive action:

■ If no test method validation exists, one must be performed before routine product testing can resume.
■ If the validated test method was not followed, retraining is in order.
■ If the SOP does not align with the validated test method, then it must be revised to bring it into alignment with laboratory practice. The rule of thumb is to "do what you say, and say what you do."

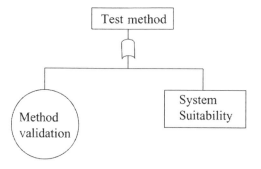

FIGURE 3

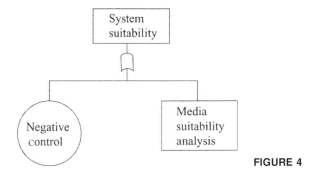

FIGURE 4

- If the analyst experienced problems with the test method, an optimization study may be in order to examine the ruggedness of the sterility test method for that product.

System Suitability
"System suitability" is the collection of controls that applies to an individual sterility test. We might identify two components of a sterility test system suitability control set: the negative control and the media suitability analyses (Fig. 4).

Negative Control
The negative control is a sterility test without a sample. Its purpose is to examine the degree of control over the aggregate of the test conditions, including the analyst's technique at the time of the test. As there is no sample involved, the rate of positives observed on the negative control provides a measure of the laboratory's or the analyst's inherent rate of "false-positives." False-positives have identifiable causes: lack of assurance of the sterility of the media, lack of assurance of the sterility of the equipment, an uncontrolled environment, and poor analyst technique are all possible causes of growth in a negative control. Therefore, when looking at an individual sterility test positive, it is important to examine the test results for the associated negative control to help determine if a systemic laboratory error (e.g., media or equipment processing, cleaning) or an analyst error (e.g., poor aseptic technique) might have occurred.

Objective evidence:

- The test record for the lot in question will document the result of the negative control. Growth in this control indicates that some component of the system was out of control on the day of the test. If so, further investigation needs to be performed to determine out where a systemic or incidental error might have occurred.
- The test record and personnel-monitoring records could indicate that the problem was associated with the analyst's technique. Identification of a "people" organism in the negative control such as *Staphylococcus epidermidis* could support the theory that there was a possible break in aseptic technique on the part of the analyst.
- The media suitability analysis record would confirm the sterility of the diluting fluid as well as the other media used in the performance of the test. If, for

example, the diluting fluid were not sterile, one would expect the negative control as well as most, if not all of the test samples that utilized that lot of diluting fluid to be positive, and to be positive with common organisms. If the analyst exhibits poor aseptic technique, one would expect that some number of his/her tests as well as some number of his/her negative controls over time would be positive, and would most likely be positive with an organism usually associated with people, e.g., *Staphylococcus or Propionibacterium*.

■ The environmental testing record will indicate the numbers and types of microorganisms isolated from the test area and will provide a measure of the control of the environment on the day of the test. High counts could suggest that either there was an intervention without sufficient cleaning (e.g., repair) or that the cleaning was ineffective and that a poorly controlled environment could have been, in part, responsible for growth in the negative control.

■ The autoclave charts will indicate if the validated times and temperatures were met for the sterilization of equipment used in the performance of the test.

■ The cleaning log will indicate if and when the area was cleaned prior to the test and who did the cleaning.

   Corrective action (or) preventive action:

■ If investigation into the history of the analyst's test results indicates that he/she has had an unusually high number of negative controls exhibiting growth in the past, then a retraining could be in order. As a note, the total number of negative controls that exhibit growth across all analysts in the laboratory using a membrane filtration (MF) manifold method under laminar flow in a cleanroom should not exceed 0.5% (16). Clearly, it would be expected that the use of isolators or closed testing systems would drive the acceptable number of false-positives much lower (Appendix 2).

■ Evidence of improperly sterilized media or equipment will invalidate all testing during that session. All media or equipment associated with the improper sterilization run must be removed from use.

■ A poor testing environment indicates a lack of control in the test area. For example, nonconforming counts under laminar flow hoods (LAFs) and biosafety cabinets could signal that maintenance and/or cleaning is in order.

Media Suitability Analysis

The USP chapter on sterility testing has a section entitled, "Suitability Tests" (4). These tests refer to the examination of each lot of bacteriological growth medium and diluting fluid used in the performance of the sterility test to assure that (i) it is sterile, (ii) it supports growth, and (iii) it has been stored properly. Not meeting the requirements of any of the suitability tests could compromise the validity of the sterility test (Fig. 5).

Media Sterility

Each lot of bacteriological growth medium, sterility test diluent, and environmental monitoring media, whether commercially prepared and purchased or prepared in-house, must undergo a preincubation to demonstrate that the lot is sterile. USP requires that a portion of each lot (unopened containers) of media used in the sterility test be incubated for 14 days to demonstrate sterility. Some laboratories preincubate the entire lot and some laboratories incubate a randomly selected

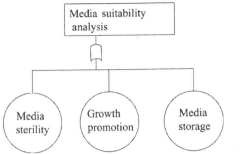

FIGURE 5

and statistically valid subset of the lot. The acceptance criterion for media sterility is that none of the incubated units exhibits growth in the 14-day period of the test. If growth is observed in this portion of the media suitability tests, the lot of medium should be rejected and must not be used in any testing.

Growth during preuse testing of a lot of purchased media indicates preparation or sterilization problems at the vendor, packaging integrity problems, or transport problems. Transport has two components with respect to purchased media. The first is transport chain between the manufacturer/distributor/customer. The second is transport within the lab from an unclassified space to a classified space or between spaces of "dirtier" to "cleaner" room classifications. A positive on a lot of medium made in-house could indicate bioburden/organism resistance problems in the dehydrated media, sterilization problems including autoclave cycle validation, storage problems, or transport problems.

Objective evidence:

■ Records of the sterility portion of the media suitability test for this lot of medium used in a sterility test including sterility media, diluting fluid, and solid media used for environmental monitoring must be complete and available for inspection.
■ Media preparation documents, sterilization charts, and storage conditions (incubator charts) must be examined carefully in the event of a positive on media prepared in-house.
■ In addition, examine the history of the media testing for past instances of positive results. Look for trends in positive results that may be related to types of media, manufacturer of the media (if purchased), manufacturer and lot number of the media powder, and sterilization records of the medium (if prepared in-house).

Corrective action (or) preventive action:

■ If media are purchased, an investigation into the lack of assurance of sterility, including a directed audit of the media manufacturer should be one outcome of a media positive. If a directed audit is called for, examine the manufacturer's processes and documentation including validation for the media preparation, packaging, sterilization, testing, storage, and transport.
■ For media prepared in-house, if deficiencies are found in preparation, sterilization, or storage, it must be determined if there was an acute problem (e.g., someone set the autoclave on the wrong cycle) or if there is a chronic problem (e.g., the autoclave cycle is inappropriate). Single instances of media failures would suggest the former; multiple instances of media failures would suggest the latter.

■ Any excursion from expected results should automatically require the quarantine of any remaining media until the results of a laboratory investigation into the deviation are analyzed, the root cause of the excursion is identified, and appropriate CAPAs are implemented.

Growth Promotion Test of Aerobes, Anaerobes, and Fungi

The second part of the USP media suitability test is meant to demonstrate that each lot of medium will support the growth of low numbers (<100 CFU) of indicator microorganisms that are identified in a USP panel of suggested organisms. The panel is the same panel recommended for the validation of the sterility test and includes a spectrum of organisms covering aerobes and anaerobes, Gram-positive and Gram-negative, spore formers and nonspore formers, bacteria and fungi, and yeast and mold. Inclusion of an environmental isolate that is not part of the USP panel is expected by some regulators to represent organisms that might be selected by conditions in the particular manufacturing environment. For example, it is appropriate to use an organism isolated from a beta-lactam manufacturing facility for test method validation and media testing because this organism is likely resistant to beta-lactam antibiotics.

Objective evidence:

■ Records of the growth-promotion suitability test must be available. Records should minimally include the date of manufacture, test date, expiration date, the types and numbers organisms (confirmed using either pour plate or MF methods) used to test each type of medium, the number of passages from the primary culture, incubation times and temperatures, confirmation that growth occurred as appropriate with the required time, and analyst initials.
■ If a supplier qualification study including a vendor audit and a product validation study has determined that a certificate of analysis from the media vendor attesting to the sterility and growth promotion of the media is acceptable, then a certificate should be on file for each lot of media or diluting fluid used in the performance or surveillance of the test. Certificates of analysis should not be accepted from the media manufacturer until proper vendor qualification and certificate verification testing has been performed and documented. Media are critical to a valid sterility test, so the vendor should be recertified on a regular basis.

Corrective action (or) preventive action:

■ Any excursion from expected results should automatically require the quarantine of any remaining media until the results of a laboratory investigation into the deviation are analyzed, the root cause of the excursion is identified, and appropriate CAPAs are implemented. Growth-promotion testing may deviate from the expected outcome for a number of reasons including but not limited to overdiluted or low-viability inoculum and dry plates.

Media Storage

The stability of any growth medium, whether purchased or prepared in-house, must be determined through validation to determine an appropriate expiration date. If a certificate of analysis for expiration date is accepted, it must be confirmed in the user laboratory. The medium must not be used if it is beyond its expiration date.

The real risk of using expired media in a sterility test is not a false-positive, but a false-negative due to the potential for "old" media not to support growth. Expiration dating is an indicator of media robustness and must be examined for a complete investigation into overall laboratory control.

Objective evidence:

■ Media suitability test records and/or certificates of analysis must be examined for evidence of expiration dating and for matching of expiration dates to testing dates.

Corrective action (or) preventive action:

■ Dispose of any media that is beyond its expiration date.

In the end, look back at the media preparation and testing records to see if the lots of media used in the OOS test had been used elsewhere, and examine those testing records for excursions or nonconformities. Patterns of excursions might indicate that a particular lot or manufacturer of media is problematic, and may require destruction of remaining units of the medium, an audit of the manufacturer, or the validation of a second supplier (Fig. 6).

ORGANISM IDENTIFICATION

Organisms isolated from any positive sterility test as well as any Class 100 (Grade A/B, ISO 5) environment, both the manufacturing and testing environments, should be identified to genus and species (1,17). There are two reasons for this:

■ The manufacturer needs to know and understand the normal flora of both the manufacturing and testing areas. Knowing the flora assists in sanitizer effectiveness studies and cleaning validation studies. Normal flora are an important source of environmental isolates to use for method validation and media testing.

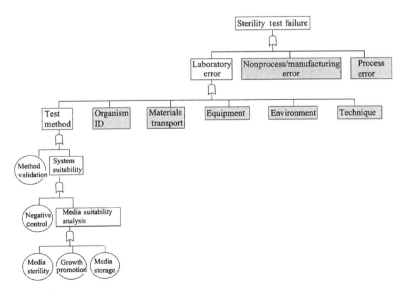

FIGURE 6

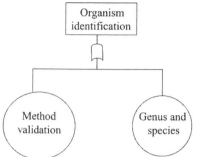

FIGURE 7

■ Matching recovered organisms from manufacturing or testing environments
with isolates recovered in the sterility test will help to answer the question,
"Was the OOS isolate also recovered from the manufacturing area, the manufacturing operators, the sterility test area, or the sterility analyst?"

When looking at the process of organism ID, one might examine two different aspects of the identification process that could affect investigation outcome, the
validation of the identification method, and the likelihood of possible sources of
the identified organism (Fig. 7).

Validation of Organism Identification Methodology

Identification can take place on pure cultures of isolates using a number of different methods including nucleic acid "fingerprint" analysis and biochemical reaction
profile (17). In any method, the identification of an isolate is determined by comparing the profile from an individual analysis to profiles contained in a broad
database of known and previously identified organisms. The result is a mathematical probability associated with a match of the unknown to an organism profile that
is contained in the database. However, databases may be built on information from
nonmanufacturing sources. For example, some databases may be built from information gathered on clinical rather than manufacturing isolates. It is important to
know and understand the source of the system's database.

Any identification method used in the laboratory must be fully validated. As
with any piece of analytical equipment, an ID system must have a documented
installation qualification (IQ), operational qualification (OQ), and performance
qualification (PQ). As part of the qualification process, a panel of known organisms, as suggested by manufacturer, must be consistently and correctly identified.

Objective evidence:

■ Executed and signed IQ, OQ, and PQ must be on file for an automated system;
method validation for a manual system.

Corrective action (or) preventive action:

■ If a system or database is deemed inappropriate for the task, a second system
must be qualified.
■ If the system has not been qualified, all the identifications from that system
are questionable. The instrument should be taken out of service and properly
validated.

Organism Identification
Once validated, the real likelihood of any identification test result must be carefully examined by the testing laboratory. For example, if the identification system suggests that the organism isolated from your sterility OOS is *Yersinia* (aka *Pasturella*) *pestis*, you should have a healthy dose of skepticism, as *Yersinia pestis* is the organism responsible for the plague in sixteenth century Europe. Although anything is possible, it is highly unlikely that this organism is the reason for your twenty-first century sterility OOS. Likewise, a saltwater marine microorganism might find its way into a facility that is located near the beach but is unlikely to be found in a Midwest manufacturing facility. When reviewing the ID of an isolate, think carefully about the foundation of the referenced database (e.g., clinical vs. industrial or environmental) and the likelihood of the isolation that organism from your manufacturing or testing environment. If you have any concerns, run the isolate through a second, validated system.

Once you are comfortable with the identification of the organism, you can use it as a clue for the rest of the investigation. For example, the recovery of *Propionibacterium acnes* from the OOS would suggest that the source of the contamination is a person or people. The investigation could focus on the people as a likely source of the contamination by looking at (i) organisms recovered from surfaces where analysts routinely touch (e.g., handles, intercoms), (ii) "touch or finger plates" that are taken routinely upon exit from the test area, and (iii) any analyst gown monitoring that might take place upon exit from the sterility test suite. Identification of *Pseudomonas* species might suggest that the source of the contamination was water, and the investigation could focus on potential leaks, quality of the WFI used in cleaning and manufacture, etc. Identification of *Pseudomonas* species as a contaminant in the product is also a clue to look for endotoxin contamination in the product and intermediates, as endotoxin is a byproduct of the growth and reproduction of Gram-negative species. If the same organism is isolated from the sample, the manufacturing environments analysts, the testing environment and manufacturing operators, the batch should be rejected unless typing using advanced nucleic acid techniques definitively eliminates manufacturing as a source of contamination (1,2,17).

Objective evidence:

- Identification documentation including a "reality check" of the probability of the isolate as identified is required. Questions to be asked include: "Is this organism part of the normal flora of this geographic area?" "Has this organism been identified in this facility before—could it possibly be part of the normal flora of the manufacturing or testing areas?" "Could people, materials, or equipment have brought this organism into the facility?"
- The laboratory's trending and database of organisms recovered in the manufacturing and testing areas will help determine the likelihood of the identification and at least circumstantial evidence as to its origin.
- Sorting OOS test results by organism or by recovery date will determine if the isolation of the organism is seasonal or if there is a correlation between organism recovered and a specific product, or a specific analyst.

Corrective action (or) preventive action:

- If the identification is unlikely, check the purity of the culture. Maybe you are identifying the wrong organism. If you are convinced that the identification is improbable, try and identify the organism on another system to confirm the ID.

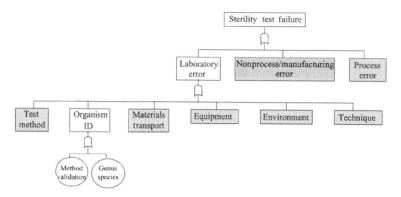

FIGURE 8

■ If trending indicates that the problem is seasonal, then validation of a change in sanitizer or cleaning regimen might be in order. For example, if *Bacillus thuringiensis* is used by the municipality in the summer for mosquito control and it is recovered seasonally in the cleanroom, then sanitizers used in the summer must demonstrate effectiveness against this organism (Fig. 8).

MATERIALS TRANSPORT

By "materials," we mean those materials, other than liquid media and sterility testing equipment, that are transported into and out of the sterility test suite for the purposes of testing. Where possible, the preferred method of materials transport into any cleanroom is via a double-door sterilizer. However, some supplies used in the performance of the sterility test are not heat stable, and therefore require a documented and validated procedure for entry into the cleanroom. Two categories of materials immediately come to mind: the test sample itself and any materials that are wrapped multiple times for the purposes of clean transport (e.g., contact plates for microbiological monitoring of the sterility test suite) (Fig. 9).

The Sterility Test Sample

One very common cause of a sterility test failure is the sample itself—not the sample material, but the outside of the sample container. It only makes sense that if one is taking precautions to keep the sterility test suite as clean as possible, then the outsides of any containers, including the sterility test sample, must be properly and

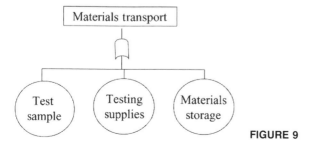

FIGURE 9

completely sanitized prior to transport into the test area. "Dunking" sealed vials or ampoules in 0.5% hypochlorite or another sporocide prior to transport into the suite is one method that is commonly used, but validation must include data to prove that sanitizer does not leak into the vials during submission. If vials come from the filling line with the plastic flip caps on them, remove the flip seals prior to sanitization. Unless validated, one cannot be certain that the sanitizer will effectively reach under the flip cap. If samples are taken in jars or plastic containers, a suitable "wipe down" procedure using an appropriate sanitizer will have to be validated.

Objective evidence:

■ A validation study of the sanitization method for bringing the samples into the area is required. Validation must include the effectiveness of the sanitization procedure against organisms commonly found in the environment.
■ An analyst interview will indicate if proper transport procedures were followed.

Corrective action (or) preventive action:

■ If a validated transport method does not exist, assure that one is developed. Ineffective sanitization of the sample is a common source of contamination that could ultimately find its way into a sterility test.

Testing Supplies

Depending on the set-up of the suite, other materials such as the heat labile parts of air samplers, the pumps used during the test, or prepared solid media used for environmental monitoring need to be transported into the test area. Prepared, purchased media are generally double- or triple-wrapped, meaning that the outermost wrapping is not sterile, but the inner wrappings are sterile. Wrappings should be removed and discarded as entry into the cleanroom progresses. Whatever the sequence, the method needs to be clearly documented in an SOP and validated. If a piece of equipment cannot be submerged or presterilized, a sequential "wipe down" procedure for exposed surfaces should be clearly documented. Under no circumstances should cardboard or laboratory papers be brought into a cleanroom. These articles are loaded with microorganisms and can be a significant source of contamination. If paper and writing implements are needed in the cleanroom, suitable autoclavable materials should be preapproved and the sterilization cycle validated before use.

Objective evidence:

■ SOPs and executed validation protocols for material transport, including sample preparation, should be examined.
■ An analyst interview should be performed to see if anything was different on the day of the test (e.g., new lot of isopropyl alcohol (IPA), change in packaging on prepared media, use of a replacement pump or air sampler that had been stored in a warehouse, lack of following the established and validated SOP, etc.).

Corrective action (or) preventive action:

■ If a validated transport method does not exist, one must be proposed and executed.
■ Validation for transport may need reexamination if it is determined that there are logistical obstacles to good practice.
■ If materials were brought into the suite improperly, any remaining materials should be removed from the area, reprocessed if possible, and the analysis retrieved.

Materials Storage

Part of material handling is the storage of the supplies and equipment once in the cleanroom. Short-term storage of media and other supplies in a cleanroom or isolator is fine provided that the environment is stable and the conditions (length of storage, temperature, humidity, and expiration date) have been determined and validated. Once asepsis is broken (e.g., shutdown, power failure, temperature or humidity excursion), any remaining test materials should be removed from the area and discarded or resanitized prior to bringing them back into the test area.

Objective evidence:

- Work orders, room temperature/humidity charts, records of differential pressures, and entry logs are all types of evidence that should be examined to assure that the materials used in the performance of the test had not been subjected to a break in asepsis.

Corrective action (or) preventive action:

- If asepsis had been broken or if it is unsure whether or not asepsis had been broken, the room must be emptied of all materials, and the materials must be discarded, resterilized, or resanitized before restocking the suite prior to resuming testing. If SOPs do not exist that outline procedures that need to be taken if asepsis is broken, they need to be written or revised so that excursions are handled consistently and properly (Fig. 10).

EQUIPMENT

All equipment used in the performance of the sterility test must be prepared and used with the focus on eliminating the possibility of contamination during the test (Fig. 11).

- Where possible, all equipment, including cleaning supplies, manifolds, punches, and forceps, should enter the cleanroom via a "pass through" sterilizer. Sterilization load patterns and cycles must be documented, validated and monitored.

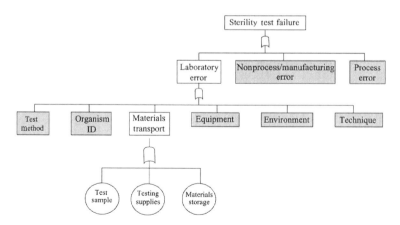

FIGURE 10

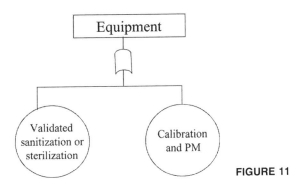

FIGURE 11

- Laminar flow hoods used in the performance of the test must be certified as Class 100 and subject to the same preventive maintenance and recertification procedures as any LFH unit used in manufacturing.
- Sanitization of the surfaces in the sterility test hood must be validated. Periodic breakdown and thorough cleaning of the hood must be validated and documented.
- Air samplers used to monitor the air for viables and nonviables during the course of the test must be calibrated and maintained in the same manner and on the same schedule as units used to monitor manufacturing. All air sampler parts must be subject to a validated sterilization or sanitization regimen.
- Manifolds and pumps used in the sterility test must be included in a detailed and documented preventive maintenance program. Any mechanical pipettors used in the performance of the test must be calibrated, and disposable tips must be sterile.
- Incubators must be qualified (IQ, OQ, and PQ). Qualification includes temperature uniformity studies. Incubators should be cleaned on a regular basis and the cleaning should be documented in the cleaning and use log for the equipment.
- Chart recorders for incubators must be subject to validation and regular calibration.

Objective evidence:

- Calibration and maintenance records must be checked to assure that all equipment used in the performance of the failed test were in good repair and in calibration. Equipment failure or unmonitored wear and tear are potential causes of a sterility test failure. For example, test failures linked to a common filtration manifold could suggest that improper sterilization of the manifold is a potential root cause of the failure.
- Sterilization records for equipment, cleaning supplies, and media for the OOS test in question must be checked to assure that the sterilization parameters were consistent with the validated cycles. Shortened cycles or lower temperatures could result in nonsterile equipment.

Corrective action (or) preventive action:

- Validated sterilization cycles must be developed if they do not exist. Cycles and loads must be revalidated regularly.
- Calibration and preventive maintenance SOPs and records must be detailed and must be available for inspection (Fig. 12).

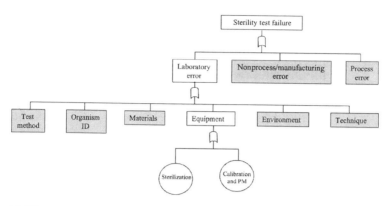

FIGURE 12

ENVIRONMENT

The drug manufacturer is required to provide an environment for testing that is at least as good as the environment used for aseptically filling the product (1,18). As the test is so labor-intensive and prone to contamination via manipulation, it makes good compliance, scientific, and financial sense to provide an environment that will limit the exposure of the product to contaminating microorganisms during the course of the test. There are two aspects to designing a stable environment for testing: (i) establishing control and (ii) monitoring as an indication of stability and maintenance of control (Fig. 13).

Establishing Control
Control is established mechanically and procedurally through:

- Good design and construction
- Thorough and complete qualification
- Validated sanitizers and cleaning procedures
- Limiting access to only those employees who are trained (Fig. 14)

Design and Construction
Sterility testing must be performed in an environment that is at least as clean as the environment used for aseptic filling (1). This means that the sterility test suite must

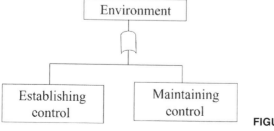

FIGURE 13

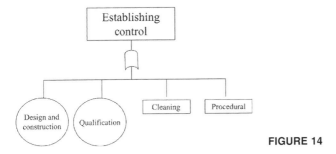

FIGURE 14

incorporate the same design elements (air velocity, air changes, differential pressures, unidirectional airflow, temperature, humidity, and surface finishes) as an aseptic filling suite.

Objective evidence:

■ The Basis of Design documents will describe the design of the cleanroom.
■ Records of work orders are an indicator of good design and construction as well as an indicator of the stability of the testing suite. Repeating problems documented in work orders may indicate design or construction problems.
■ Temperature, humidity, and differential pressure records may suggest trends or patterns that are indicators of environmental instability of the area. Recurring or chronic excursions in any of these areas may be an indicator of poor design and/or construction.

Corrective action (or) preventive action:

■ A poorly designed and poorly maintained sterility test suite is an OOS sterility test waiting to happen. Every effort must be made to design and maintain an environment that will minimize the possibility of extrinsic test contamination. If the testing area is poorly designed, consideration should be given to shutting the area down, redesigning the suite to at least filling suite specifications, and requalifying it accordingly.

Qualification
Just as an aseptic filling suite, the sterility test suite must be fully qualified, including a properly executed and documented IQ and OQ, and a PQ. For isolators, initial qualification includes an IQ, an OQ, and a PQ as described by the manufacturer and as outlined in USP (19). Qualification serves a number of purposes, among them confirmation of the direction and velocity of the airflow, differential pressure between contiguous rooms, determination of a nonviable particulate count consistent with EU, ISO, or USP standards, identification of a "baseline" microbiological flora in the area, the effectiveness of cleaning, and the ability to choose appropriate sampling sites based on microbial recovery patterns.

Objective evidence:

■ Validation documents will describe the qualification specifications and acceptance criteria for the sterility test area and/or isolator. For a sterility testing suite, the validation parameters and acceptance criteria must be equal to or better than the filling suite.

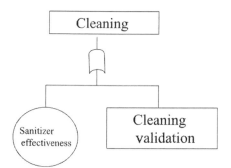

FIGURE 15

Corrective action (or) preventive action:

■ If it is found that the suite was not qualified, the room must be shut down, and properly qualified in order to bring it back into compliance.

Cleaning
There are two aspects to cleaning control: the initial selection of appropriate and effective sanitizers and validation of the cleaning procedure (Fig. 15).

Sanitizer Effectiveness
Sanitizers must be chosen for their effectiveness against a known panel of organisms, as well as organisms isolated from the manufacturing and testing environments (1). The effectiveness of rotation of sanitizers is a matter of some discussion among those in the industry, but whatever sanitization regimen is used it must be validated to be effective on a spectrum of microorganisms including mold and bacterial spores across all seasons of the year. Validation includes in vitro experiments such as the Association of Official Agricultural Chemists Use Dilution Test (20) and a determination that contaminating microorganisms will be removed effectively from all surfaces and finishes during cleaning. These studies must ultimately define sanitizer concentration, contact time, cleaning frequency, the sterility of the sanitizer or process by which sanitizers are rendered sterile, and effective rinsing processes for the elimination of sanitizer residuals (21,22).

Objective evidence:

■ Examination of sanitizer effectiveness validation data and comparison with isolates from the environment and failed sterility test will determine if the sanitizers used are effective against the organisms that are recovered from the area.
■ Examination of microbiological monitoring data from the area after cleaning and prior to testing may suggest that sanitizers and/or cleaning techniques are ineffective. Upward trends in microbiological monitoring data that can be associated with a change in cleaning solutions, tools, regimen, or crews may suggest a problem.

Corrective action (or) preventive action:

■ Trending high microbial counts could warrant a number of additional actions including conducting sanitizer effectiveness studies on environmental isolates, retraining of cleaning crew, and reexamination of preparation of sanitizers, and sterilization of cleaning equipment.

Cleaning Validation

A successful cleaning validation requires attention to three important functions. The first is sanitizer effectiveness (above). The second is the definition of proper cleaning technique and the third is training in proper cleaning. The technique must take into account equipment, chemical nature of the sanitizer, sanitizer concentration, contact time, and cleaning sequence methodology (top to bottom of the room and far side of the room to the door) (Fig. 16).

Cleaning validation is often incorporated into the PQ of the cleanroom. Cleaning validation has two parts: demonstration of the stability of the environment under static conditions, and the continued ability of the cleaning regimen to maintain stability of the environment under dynamic conditions. Instability in the environment under PQ may suggest problems with the cleaning validation protocol, the sanitizer effectiveness, the frequency of cleaning, equipment, or cleaning methods.

Objective evidence:

- Cleaning logs will tell you who cleaned, when he/she/they cleaned, and how long it took to clean the area.
- Autoclave logs and charts will tell you what equipment and solutions (including water) were sterilized for cleaning. Note: concentrated sanitizers, if not received as sterile, should be filter-sterilized prior to use.
- Training records of cleaners will tell you if the cleaning crew is trained in the most recent SOP.

Corrective action (or) preventive action:

- Incomplete records such as entry logs, cleaning logs, and autoclave chart annotation will require retraining in proper documentation.
- Improper sterilization of equipment will require revalidation of sterilization runs.
- If cleaning sessions are considerably shorter or longer than expected, retraining may be in order. Short cleaning sessions may suggest an incomplete cleaning session. Long cleaning sessions may suggest that a problem was encountered during the session.
- If training records suggest that cleaners are new to the job, or have not been to a cleaning refresher course, it could be time to schedule one.

Procedure

Establishing and maintaining control of cleanrooms is supported by a level of procedural control (Fig. 17).

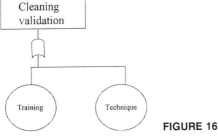

FIGURE 16

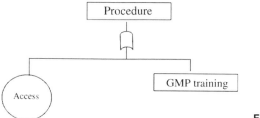

FIGURE 17

Access

Access to sterility test areas must be limited to those who have specific training in their assigned cleanroom tasks. Only trained cleaners should have access to the area for cleaning. Only trained sterility test analysts should have access to the area during testing. Everyone with access to the suite, including mechanics and engineers, must be trained in gowning, GMPs, basic microbiology, and cleanroom etiquette. Visitors who have a specific purpose such as repair in the area must be accompanied at all times through gowning and completion of their task. Unscheduled visits to the cleanroom by anyone other than analysts or cleaners should be followed by a thorough cleaning. A break in asepsis for the purposes of repair must be followed by the same multiple cleaning regimen that would be used in the aseptic manufacturing area.

Objective evidence:

- Entry logs must be checked for unauthorized access to sterility testing areas prior to the session where the OOS result occurred.
- Cleaning logs must be checked to assure that any unusual access (e.g., repair) was followed by a thorough cleaning.
- Cleaning logs must also be checked to assure that the area was sanitized prior to testing, either earlier in the day or the evening before. Unauthorized or unscheduled activity without cleaning may have caused a break in asepsis, which could have contributed to the OOS. The environmental-monitoring profile will indicate whether or not a break in asepsis has occurred.

Corrective action (or) preventive action:

- If examination of entry and cleaning logs indicate that there was unusual activity in the area that was not followed by an extensive cleaning, the area must be shut down and resanitized.

GMP Training

A rigorous training program is the cornerstone of a well-controlled area (Fig. 18) (23).

Cleanroom Etiquette

All people working in a cleanroom must understand that behavior affects cleanliness. Even when gowned, people shed particles and microorganisms. Requiring that jewelry and make up be removed before entering the area controlling movements once in the area and attention to frequent disinfection of hands are but three components of good cleanroom behavior.

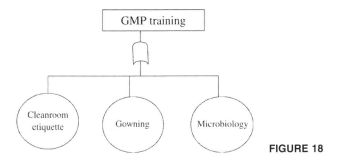

FIGURE 18

Gowning
All people entering the sterility test suite (analysts, cleaners, mechanics) must be properly gowned for work in aseptic areas. However, work at an isolator requires no special gowning. Proper gowning requires extensive training and certification.

Education
As part of GMP training, all cleanroom personnel, including sterility test analysts, should learn the basic principles of microbiology. They should know where organisms come from, how they are transported to and deposited in the cleanroom, how microbiological contamination is detected, and how it is prevented (1).

Objective evidence:

- Training records will indicate deficiencies in training and/or a need for recertification.
- Personnel monitoring data for anyone entering the area will indicate any upward trends in counts of all people entering the area.
- Records of periodic observation of the sterility test analyst by supervisory staff may reveal behaviors or techniques that could result in a break in asepsis.

Corrective action (or) preventive action:

- Upward trends in personnel monitoring will require retraining.
- Observed behaviors that could result in contamination of the sterility test will require retraining (Fig. 19).

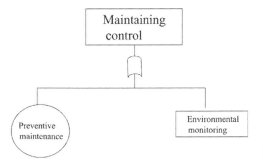

FIGURE 19

Maintaining Control

Preventive Maintenance

A significant factor in the maintenance of the cleanroom is the preventive maintenance of the HVAC system. As with the manufacturing area, high-efficiency
particulate air (HEPA) filters in the sterility test cleanroom must be qualified upon
installation and recertified periodically and the air flow and differential pressure
between rooms must be balanced.

Objective evidence:

■ Equipment log books or electronic preventive maintenance logs and equipment stickers must be checked to assure that calibration and preventive
maintenance is current.

Corrective action (or) preventive action:

■ If any equipment is found to be out of calibration or is found to be beyond its
scheduled preventive maintenance, it should be taken out of service until the
calibration or service is performed.
■ If equipment (e.g., the LFH, the autoclave, the HEPA filters) is found to be out
of calibration or beyond its preventive maintenance timepoint, check previous
testing back to the piece's last calibration or preventive maintenance to look for
patterns or trends in nonconforming results that used that piece of equipment
(Fig. 20).

Environmental Monitoring

Once control is established through proper specifications, design, qualification,
and procedure, control is maintained through careful and thoughtful environmental monitoring (14,18). Temperature, humidity, and differential pressure must be
monitored continuously. An increase in temperature and/or humidity may change
conditions sufficiently to support bacterial and mold growth. In addition, an
increase in temperature and/or humidity makes conditions uncomfortable for
the analyst, perhaps increasing perspiration inside the sterile gown. Increasing perspiration increases the possibility of contamination. The sterility test suite must be
under positive pressure relative to the adjacent rooms. A change in differential
pressure and at the extreme, a change from positive to negative pressure, could
allow organisms in the air from adjacent less clean areas to stream into the testing
area (Fig. 21).

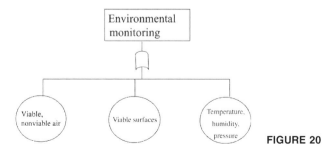

FIGURE 20

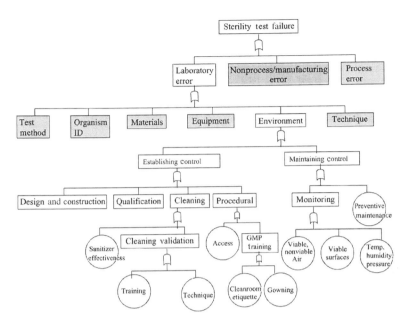

FIGURE 21

Monitoring of air for viable and nonviable particulates as well as monitoring of surfaces for evidence of viables is expected (1). Just as in an aseptic processing area, there are six kinds of monitoring that must take place:

1. The surfaces are monitored with contact plates after cleaning but prior to testing as a check on the effectiveness of the routine cleaning. The ability of the neutralizers contained in the contact plates to inactivate residual sanitizers must be validated. If neutralizers do not successfully inactivate the sanitizer, counts that are observed in routine monitoring may be falsely depressed. If inactivation is unsuccessful, changes to the cleaning regimen, the sanitizers, and/or the neutralizers may be in order.
2. Monitoring surfaces after testing will provide data on the "cleanliness" of the testing operation.
3. Monitoring of the air for viables and nonviables before the test will provide an indication of the stability of the test environment.
4. Monitoring the air for viables and nonviables during the test provides information on the "cleanliness" of the immediate testing environment.
5. Monitoring the air for nonviable particulates is a check on alignment with USP and ISO nonviable particle requirements for classified cleanrooms.
6. A major source of contamination both in manufacturing and in testing is the operator. We have "one shot" at a sterility test, and it is important to demonstrate that the analyst can keep the test clean. One method of monitoring the analyst is through personnel monitoring, i.e., the use of contact plates to look for microbial contamination on the hands and on the gown.

The process for choosing monitoring sites and frequencies in the sterility test suite should mirror the process used for manufacturing. At a minimum, the suite needs to be monitored on each testing day and each testing session during the day, and the analyst needs to be monitored at the close of each testing session.

High counts in the testing suite and a genus/species match between organisms recovered in the failed test and in the test area may provide support for the invalidation of the sterility test (1,17). However, the justification cannot be made in the absence of data from manufacturing areas and operators. For example, if an organism is found on the sterility test analyst, in the sterility test area, and in the aseptic core (not even the specific rooms where manufacture or filling of the lot in question took place), one cannot rule out the possibility that the contamination came from the manufacturing area.

Objective evidence:

■ Records of temperature, humidity, and differential pressure should be available in the laboratory. Charts from recorders should be changed, reviewed, and signed by trained analysts who will be able to immediately spot excursions. If temperature, humidity, and pressure are monitored through an electronic building maintenance system (BMS), records should be checked for the frequency and extent of excursions with an eye toward looking for patterns or trends that could adversely affect the environment.
■ Environmental-monitoring records consisting of viable and nonviable air data, viable surface data, and personnel monitoring must be examined. In addition to data from the date and session in question, monitoring data from before and after the OOS date need to be examined for trends or patterns in quantitative or qualitative recovery of organisms or nonviable counts.
■ Personnel monitoring records will indicate whether the analyst exceeded limits on the day of the test, and what types of organisms were recovered. These identified organisms must be compared to the OOS recovered organism.
■ Preventive maintenance records for the area must be checked to see if unusual activity was evident in the room that might have resulted in a contamination event.

Corrective action (or) preventive action:

■ An upward trend in environmental monitoring data (viable and/or nonviable) suggests that the area is out of control. Looking at cleaning, work orders, entry logs, certification reports, etc. may provide clues as to the types of preventive and corrective actions that need to occur. Some of these actions may be as simple as a filter replacement or limiting access, while others, like correcting poor technique or cleanroom behavior, might take considerably more thought and effort (Fig. 21).

TECHNIQUE

Sterility, by definition, is an absolute. We are required to make and test sterile products in an aseptic environment, which is very clean, but because it is inhabited by people, it is not sterile. In spite of all of our efforts to control environmental conditions of the test through design, construction, sanitization, gowning, and HEPA-filtered air, the outcome of the sterility test is remarkably dependent on the analyst's aseptic technique (Fig. 22).

In theory, there should never be a sterility test positive on a terminally sterilized (TS) product. A positive indicates one of the two things: an inadequately sterilized product or contamination during testing. Assuming a validated sterilization

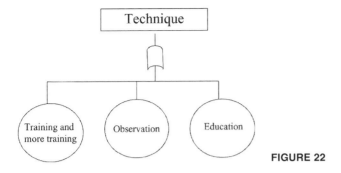

FIGURE 22

cycle and no deviations in the manufacture of the product, the most likely reason for a positive on a TS product is the analyst. Having said that, the investigation into a TS-positive must be as complete, scientific, and unbiased to provide objective evidence to justify any thoughts of invalidation of the test result.

Training, Education, and Observation

The appropriate level of education and extensive training is essential to a good outcome in a sterility test. If analysts are not trained microbiologists, they should undergo training to learn and understand what microorganisms are, where they come from, how they find their way into the product, how to keep them out of a sterility test, and the compliance and financial consequences of a sterility test failure.

Manipulation of the test apparatus is difficult, and this manipulation, even with gloved hands working under a Class 100 LFH, can be a source of contamination. Given the difficulties, analysts should practice preparing the sample and using the apparatus first in the laboratory on a bench without worrying about asepsis. The next step is to learning work within the restricted space of a laminar flow good. Finally, gowning adds yet another restriction in movement, so practicing in the laboratory, under an LFH, while gowned is the final step before practicing in the cleanroom.

Analysts should demonstrate on terminally sterilized and noninterfering materials (e.g., WFI or microbiological growth medium in vials) that they can prepare the test sample, keep it sterile, and come out with an uncontaminated test. Once they demonstrate proficiency out of the cleanroom, then they must demonstrate proficiency in the cleanroom environment. All sterility test analysts, including the most seasoned veteran, should be observed periodically to detect breaks in acceptable aseptic technique or indications of poor cleanroom behavior.

Analysts should be trained to document all deviations to a test protocol and to terminate the procedure for all tests with clear deviations in technique that could result in a false-positive (e.g., dropping a filter, inadvertently touching a test critical surface). Attention to changes in facility, environment, test method, or technique could all be indicators of potential problems that, if corrected, could prevent a sterility OOS (1).

Objective Evidence:

■ Job descriptions will outline the education and experience expected of a sterility test analyst.

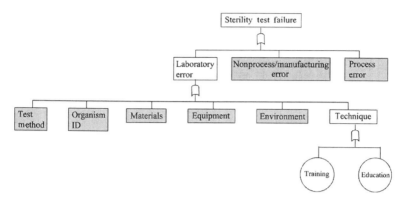

FIGURE 23

- Analyst training records will indicate the extent of training and/or experience that the analyst has had.
- Records of past OOS and false-positive results sorted by analyst will provide analyst-specific data on possible problems with technique.
- Observation records of sterility analysts provide a continuing check on technique.

    Corrective action (or) preventive action:

- There should be no hesitation on retraining for an analyst whose performance, even if not proven conclusively, suggests a problem.
- Depending on the trends/patterns in OOS data, adjustments could be made in the testing regimen. For example, if more OOS results are found toward the end of the day, every effort should be made to schedule sterility tests early in the day when analysts are fresh and alert. If analyst technique is threatened because of logistics in the testing area, an analysis of furniture placement, ergonomics, and supply storage could be examined. The idea is to make testing as easy and convenient for the analyst as possible to avoid confusion and clutter and disruption in the test area (Fig. 23).

THE CHECKLIST

By going through the preliminary work and then drilling down the fault tree through intermediate events and identifying basic events of the that could have contributed to the failure, we can create a checklist that might be used to objectively guide an investigation into a sterility test positive. The data provided in the checklist must be interpreted by the laboratory manager, and a narrative must be provided explaining if a problem was noted in the lab and if so, was the problem such that it could be a candidate for invalidating the sterility test result. The laboratory data will be considered along with the data gathered from the investigation of the manufacturing environment and process as well as all of the trend histories to determine if, in fact, the documented laboratory problem was the only identified root cause of the positive and the test can be justifiably invalidated (Table 3 & 4).

TABLE 3 Checklist for Investigation of a Sterility Test Positive

Item	Evidence	Conforms	Does not conform	Comments— comment is required for any point that "does not conform"
Product				
What is the history of OOS with this product?	Microbiology laboratory testing and trending records			
Has there been a recent change history for this product (process, formulation, change in raw material supplier)?	Change control records			
Were the appropriate number of samples tested?	Test record			
Were samples prepared and transported into the suite in the usual and appropriate manner?	Test record, analyst interview			
Analyst				
What is the history of OOS for this analyst?	Microbiology laboratory testing and trending records			
When was the last OOS for this analyst?	Microbiology laboratory testing and trending records			
Is there a correlation between positives for this product and this analyst?	Microbiology laboratory testing and trending records			
What is the history of false-positives (growth on the negative control) for this analyst?	Microbiology laboratory testing and trending records			
Test method				
Is this test method valid?	Validation records			
Was the test method followed?	Test record, analyst interview			
Were there any problems noted with preparing the sample?	Test record, analyst interview			
Were there any problems noted performing this test?	Test record, analyst interview			
Did the negative control exhibit growth?	Test record			
Media				
Were all media used in the performance of the test or in the surveillance of the test sterile?	Media preparation and testing records			

(Continued)

TABLE 3 Checklist for Investigation of a Sterility Test Positive (*Continued*)

Item	Evidence	Conforms	Does not conform	Comments—comment is required for any point that "does not conform"
Did all of the media used in the performance of the test or in the surveillance of the test support growth?	Media preparation and testing records			
Were all media used in the performance of the test or in the surveillance of the test within their expiration period?	Media preparation and testing records			
Have there been previous problems with these lots of media?	Media preparation and testing records			
Organism identification				
Is the identification method validated?	Validation records			
Has this organism been isolated from this product before?	Microbiology laboratory testing and trending records			
Was this organism isolated from the sterility test area on or around this test date?	Environmental monitoring records (sterility test area)			
Was this organism isolated from the manufacturing area on or around the manufacturing dates?	Environmental monitoring records (manufacturing area)			
Was this organism isolated from the analyst who performed the sterility test?	Personnel monitoring records			
Facilities				
Was there an interruption in power during the test?	Facilities			
Differential pressure OK?	Differential pressure monitoring			
HEPA filters certified?	Facilities			
Unscheduled maintenance required?	Work orders, entry log			
Cleaning performed as required?	Entry log, autoclave charts			
Environment				
Viable air counts on the day of the test OK?	Environmental monitoring records			

(*Continued*)

TABLE 3 Narrative: Acronyms and Definitions of Microbiological Terms (*Continued*)

Item	Evidence	Conforms	Does not conform	Comments— comment is required for any point that "does not conform"
Viable air counts for at least a month before and since the test. Any upward trends?	Environmental monitoring records			
Viable surface counts on the day of the test OK?	Environmental monitoring records			
Viable surface counts for at least a month before and since the test—any upward trends?	Environmental monitoring records			
Organism(s) isolated from the testing environment the same as isolated from the product?	Environmental monitoring records			
Nonviable counts OK?	Environmental monitoring records			
Temperature and humidity OK?	Chart recorders, BMS			
Has the operator been properly trained?	Training records			
Has the operator's technique been observed lately?	Training records			

Abbreviations: OOS, out-of-specification; EM, environmental monitoring.

TABLE 4 Narrative: Acronyms and Definitions of Microbiological Terms

Aerobe	Organisms that require oxygen to survive
Anaerobe	Organisms that can only grow in the absence of oxygen
CFU	Colony-forming units
Facultative anaerobe	Can grow in the absence or presence of oxygen
Gram-positive and gram-negative organisms	Organisms are divided into two broad categories based on their reaction in a differential staining technique called the Gram stain; differentiation is based on the ability to take up and retain a stain or counterstain based on the organism's cell wall composition
Spore (bacterial)	Sometimes called an endospore, a spore is an ovoid body formed in the vegetative cells of some gram-positive bacilli that are resistant to heat, drying, freezing, deleterious chemicals, and radiation
Spore (fungal)	Sometimes called conidia, fungal spores form singly or in clusters at the end of the hyphae found on some colonies; individual spores can separate from the fungal colony, and can be carried to a new site where, if conditions are optimum, it can germinate to form a new mold colony

Source: From Ref. 24.

REFERENCES

1. U.S. Department of Health and Human Services, Food and Drug Administration, Center for Drug Evaluation and Research (CDER), Center for Biologics Evaluation and Research (CBER), Office of Regulatory Affairs (ORA). Guidance for Industry Sterile Drug Products Produced by Aseptic Processing—Current Good Manufacturing Practice, 2004. http://www.fda.gov/cder/guidance/1874dft.doc.
2. Cundell AM. Microbial testing in support of aseptic processing. Pharmaceut Technol 2004; 56.
3. U.S. Department of Health and Human Services, Food and Drug Administration. Human Drug CGMP Notes, 1999.
4. United States Pharmacopeia 29, 2006 <71> Sterility Test.
5. United States of America, Plantiff 15 Barr Laboratories Inc, et al, Defendants Civic Action 92–1744.
6. US Department of Health and Human services. Guidance for Industry Investigations out of Specification (OOS) list Results for pharmaceutical Production, 1998.
7. Avallone HL. Sterility retesting. J Parenter Sci Technol 1986; 40(2):56–57.
8. Lee J. Investigating sterility test failures. Pharmaceut Technol 1990; 14(2):38–43.
9. U.S. Food and Drug Administration. 1997. Hazard Analysis and Critical Control Point Principles and Application Guidelines.
10. Stamatis, D. H. Failure Mode and Effect Analysis: FMEA from Theory to execution. Chapter 2: FMEA: A General Overview. ASQ Quality Press, 1993: 21–81.
11. McDermott, Robine E, Mikulak RE, Beauregard MR. The Basics of FMEA. Productivity Inc., Portland: Oregon, 1996: 27–45.
12. Vesely WE, Goldberg FF, Roberts NH, Haasl DF. Fault Tree Handbook. Washington, DC: U.S. Government Printing Office, 1981.
13. Rooney JJ, Vanden Heuvel LN. Root cause analysis for beginners. Qual Progr 2004; 45.
14. United States Pharmacopeia 29. <1227>, Validation of Microbial Recovery from Pharmacopeial Articles, 2006.
15. United States Pharmacopeia 29. <1116>, Microbiological evaluation of clean rooms and other controlled environments, 2006.
16. U.S. Department of Health Human Services, Food and Drug Administration. Aseptic Processing Guideline, 1987.
17. Sutton SVW, Cundell AM. Microbial Identification in the Pharmaceutical Industry. Stinumi to the Revision Process, United States Pharmacopeial Convention 1884–1894, 2004.
18. Deschenes P. Viable environmental microbiological monitoring: microbiology of sterilization processes. In: Frederick JC, Agalloco JP, eds. Validation of Pharmaceutical Processes. 2nd ed. New York: Marcel Dekker, 1999.
19. United States Pharmacopeia 29. <1208>, Sterility Testing—Validation of Isolator Systems, 2006.
20. AOAC Official Methods of Analysis. 17th ed., Chapter 6. Disinfectants. AOAC International, 2000 Washington DC.
21. Denney VF, Kopis EM, Marsik FJ. Elements for a successful disinfection program in the pharmaceutical environment. J Parenter Sci Technol 1999; 53(3)115–124.
22. Kaiser H, Klein D, Kopis E, LeBlanc D, McDonnell G, Tirey JF. Interaction of disinfectant residues on cleanroom substrates. J Parenter Sci Technol 1999; 53(4).
23. Dixon, AM. Training Cleanroom Personnel. J Parenter Sci Technol 1991; 45(6).
24. Davis BD, Dulbecco R, Eisen HN, Ginsberg HS, Barry Wood W. Microbiology. New York: Harper & Row, 1967.

25. Sandle T. Environmental Monitoring in a Sterility Testing Isolator, 2003. http://www.pharmig.org.uk/pages/articles/envmon.html.
26. Millipore Corporation. Steritest® User Guide, 2004. http://www.millipore.com/userguides.nsf/docs/p36200.
27. Friedman R, Mahoney SC. Risk factors in aseptic processing. Am Pharmaceut Rev 2003.
28. Leahy TJ, Roche KL, Christopher MR. Microbiology of sterilization processes. In: Carleton FJ, Agalloco JP, eds. Validation of Pharmaceutical Processes, 2nd ed. New York: Marcel Dekker, 1999.
29. International Standards Organization ISO 14644-1 "Cleanrooms and Associated Controlled Environment. Part 1: Classification of Air Cleanliness.

APPENDIX 1: THE STERILITY TEST—BIG MOVING PARTS

USP General Chapter 71, "Sterility Tests," provides the parenteral industry with clear guidelines on how to perform the sterility test and how to interpret the results (4). This USP chapter, recently harmonized philosophically with the European Pharmacopeia and the Japanese Pharmacopeia, divides the sterility test into its component parts.

Methodology

Membrane Filtration
The method of choice for the sterility test is the membrane filtration (MF) method. For this method, the analyst aseptically pools the contents of a prescribed number of containers in a volume of sterile diluting fluid. The number of units tested is taken randomly to represent the beginning, middle, and end of the batch as well as any significant interventions that happened during the course of the fill. The number of containers and the quantity of material to be tested depends on the amount of material/unit and the number of filled units in the batch as described in Tables 5 and 6 USP <71> (4).

Once the contents of the individual test units and pooled and dissolved (in the case of solids), the sample is passed through a filter with a pore size not greater than 0.45 m. After the sample has passed through the filter, it is rinsed with additional volumes of diluting fluid to rid the filter of any interfering substances (refer to "Validation"). After the final rinse, the filter is cut into two parts. One part of the cut filter is added to Soybean-Casein digest (SCD) medium and incubated for 14 days at 22.5 ± 2.5°C to provide an optimum environment for the growth of aerobic bacteria, molds, and fungi. The other part of the filter is added to fluid thioglycollate medium (FTM) and is incubated for 14 days at 32.5 ± 2.5°C

TABLE 5 Probability of a Positive Sterility Test as Function of Contamination Rate

Contamination rate	Probability of finding at least one contaminated vial in a 20 unit sample (%)
1/1000	1.9
1/500	3.9
1/200	9.5
1/100	18.2
1/50	33
1/25	55.7
1/10	87.8

to provide an optimum environment for the growth of obligate and facultative anaerobes, as well as many aerobic microorganisms. Tubes are examined periodically during this 14-day incubation period and at the end of incubation by a trained analyst to look for increasing turbidity, which is evidence of microbial growth. If no growth is observed over the 14-day incubation period, the sample, and by extension, the lot of product under test complies with the test for sterility. If growth is observed in either medium, the sample, and by extension, lot of product does not meet the requirements of the sterility test and the entire lot is subject to quarantine, investigation, and perhaps rejection.

Negative Control
The analyst prepares the negative control by performing the entire test process including filtration, rinses, filter cutting, and incubation in the absence of a test sample. This control is usually performed before the rest of the test samples are prepared and filtered to assure that conditions are optimum for a negative test, i.e., the analyst is "fresh," the testing equipment is untouched and has not been exposed to the test material, and the testing bench is impeccably clean. Negative controls are incubated and examined for the presence of growth along with the associated test articles. As no sample is involved, growth in the negative control indicates clearly that something or a combination of things in the laboratory, either the analyst, the equipment, the environment, and/or the media, could have been responsible for the contamination. Examining the number of positive responses on this control over time provides an indication of the inherent "false-positive" rate of the sterility test in the laboratory and provides a benchmark against which laboratory and testing control is measured.

Environment
Given the potential financial implications of a positive result, every effort must be taken to limit the risk of contamination during the course of the sterility test. One possible source of contamination is the testing environment.

Facilities—The Sterility Test Suite
Many companies perform sterility tests in a "sterility testing suite." The suite is a series of rooms, with appropriate gowning facilities, that mimics the production facility in its design, construction, preventive maintenance, and environmental monitoring surveillance program.

   The testing laboratory environment should employ facilities and controls comparable to those used for filling and closing operations. Poor or deficient sterility test facilities or controls can result in a high rate of test failures (1).

   What does this mean? In the case of a sterility test suite, this means:

- The sterility suite is subject to the same design elements (e.g., air velocity, air changes, differential pressures, unidirectional air flow) as the filling suite.
- The sterility suite must meet ISO 5 requirements for the immediate testing environment (LAF, biosafety cabinet) and at least ISO 7 for the space immediately adjacent to the testing environment.
- The sterility suite is subject to the same IQ, OQ, and PQ acceptance criteria as is the filling suite.
- The sterility suite is subject to the same maintenance procedures (e.g., periodic filter certification and air balancing) as the filling suite.

- Hoods or biosafety cabinets used in the suite are subject to the same qualification and maintenance procedures as the hoods used in manufacturing.
- The sterility suite is subject to the same sanitization procedures (i.e., choice and rotation of validated sanitizers, cleaning method, and cleaning frequency) as the filling suite.
- The sterility suite is subject to the same type of restricted access as the filling suite. Analysts working in the sterility suite are subject to the same gowning training and qualification/requalification requirements as operators working in the filling suite.
- The sterility suite must be monitored (viable and nonviable air and viable surface) with the same intensity and frequency as the filling suite (15). SOPs must exist for the identification of monitoring sites and frequencies in the sterility test suite. Alert and action limits, comparable to those used in manufacturing, must be documented (1,18).
- Analysts working in the sterility suite are subject to the same intensive GMP training and personnel monitoring as operators working in the aseptic manufacturing areas.

Sterility Testing Isolators

As an alternative to a sterility test suite, firms may choose to perform sterility testing in an isolator. An isolator is a carefully controlled, self-contained microenvironment. Isolators can be constructed from a number of different materials including flexible plastics, rigid–plastic, glass, or stainless steel. Air is supplied through HEPA filters, but unlike sterility suites, there is no requirement for air velocity or air exchange rate. The isolator is positive to the surrounding environment, so small leaks or pinholes in the unit, while a concern, should not allow contamination to enter. Pressure gauges monitor the pressure differential between the isolator and the surrounding environment. The interior of the isolator must meet ISO 5 conditions at rest, but there are no USP specifications for operational isolators. The unit and transfer modules must be capable of withstanding sterilization and they must be monitored (19,25). The isolator is subject to a number of extensive qualification procedures including integrity checks, sterilization cycle verification (i.e., type, concentration, and distribution of sterilant), sterilization frequency, cleaning qualification (remember, cleaning and sanitizing are two different events), and demonstration that when exposed to sterilant, the materials stored within the isolator are not compromised. The transfer of materials into and out of the isolator must be validated.

When using an isolator for sterility testing, the analyst does not handle materials or samples directly. Instead, the equipment and materials used in the sterility test are housed inside the isolator, and the analyst performs the test using gloved hands that are part of a half-suit. As neither the operator nor the laboratory environment contacts testing equipment or samples, it is expected that the use of a validated isolator will reduce or eliminate extrinsic contamination of the sterility test.

Equipment

Membrane Filtration Manifold—"Open" System

A sterility test manifold is a reusable stainless steel support for a number of covered and sterilizable filter funnels. The assembled manifold is sterilized using a validated moist heat sterilization cycle, and is placed directly under the LFH in the sterility test suite after sterilization. Filters are either sterilized in place on the manifold apparatus, or the analyst uses impeccable aseptic technique to remove each funnel and place a presterilized filter membrane on each funnel support. Introduction of diluent to wet the membrane and provide rinses for individual tests is controlled through a series of hoses and stopcocks. Sample and rinse are drawn through the filter via vacuum. After filtration and rinsing, the analyst uses a pair of sterile forceps to remove the filter from under the funnel and either cuts it or places it into a stainless steel "punch" to create two pieces—one incubated in SCD and one incubated in FTM (above). The MF test using a manifold apparatus is often referred to as an "open" system because samples and filters are exposed multiple times to the environment under the hood and are potentially subject to contamination because of the high degree of manipulation of the sample and the apparatus required of the analyst.

Membrane Filtration—"Closed" System
Alternatively, one can perform the sterility test using a "closed" system (26). The closed system contains a number of component parts—a sample preparation bottle complete with a cap and rubber septum and containing sterile diluent, sterile tubing with a sterile needle and vent at one end which splits into two tubes, each with a sterile plastic canister at the other end, a pump, and a vacuum source. Each sterile canister is fitted with a 0.45 μm filter. After sample preparation, the vented needle assembly is inserted through the septum of the sample preparation bottle. Using the pump provided in the apparatus, the prepared sample is pumped from the bottle, through the tubing, and is split equally through the two tubing pathways and through the canisters. Rinsing of the filters is accomplished in a similar manner using a bottle of sterile diluting fluid. After rinsing, the outlet of each canister is plugged to allow for the addition of growth medium. One of the tubing pathways is clamped off and SCD is pumped into one canister. After the addition of this medium, the pathway to that canister is clamped, and FTM is pumped into the remaining canister. The tubing is cut using sterile scissors, and canisters are ready for incubation. The system is called a "closed" system because the test, except for sample prep, is contained and closed to the environment (26).

Test Interpretation
USP is very clear (4):

- If no evidence of microbial growth is found, the product to be examined complies with the test for sterility.
- If evidence of microbial growth is found, the product to be examined does not comply with the test for sterility, unless it can be clearly demonstrated that the test was invalid for causes unrelated to the product to be examined.

What constitutes an invalid test? USP gives some examples, but we must recognize that these examples must be considered in the context of the overall investigation. Remember that finding of problems in both the test area and the manufacturing area assumes problems in manufacturing and defaults to a product failure. The four examples provided in USP include:

1. The data of the microbiological monitoring of the sterility testing facility show a fault.

This statement means that there is a clear and documented problem with the environment (as measured by microbiological monitoring) in the sterility test facility and there is no observed problem with the environment in the manufacturing area during either the manufacturing or the filling of the product. If there is a microbiological problem (including personnel monitoring) in both places, or if there is a problem with the sterility environment and there was any other condition during manufacture that could affect the environment (e.g., temperature or humidity spike during manufacturing or the same organism found in a different part of the aseptic manufacturing facility), then the documented problem in the lab cannot stand on its own and cannot be considered sufficient to justify invalidation of the test.

2. A review of the testing procedure used during the test in question reveals a fault.

This means that there is a documented problem with the test itself. However, if there was an obvious issue during the performance of the test, the procedure should have been stopped at that point, documented, and the tubes/canisters never should have been incubated. However, if a cap comes loose and falls off during the reading of the tubes containing the filters or if the tubing disconnects from the sterility canister and a positive is observed subsequent to that event, the test may be a candidate for invalidation provided that there are no problems associated with manufacturing.

3. Microbial growth is found in the negative controls.

A finding of growth in the negative control is indicative of a break in aseptic technique or a problem with the equipment or media. It might be reasonable to invalidate all tests referencing a nonconforming negative but one cannot pick and choose. For example, if *S. epidermidis* is found in the negative control and is also found in the SCD medium of one sample tested during that same session, how can you "clearly demonstrate" that the organism in both tubes came from the sterility operator? To make things more complicated, if *S. epidermidis* was found on one of the manufacturing operators, how can you "clearly demonstrate" that the *S. epidermidis* found in the test sample was the result of a contamination event by the sterility operator and not a contamination event by the manufacturing operator?

4. After determination of the identity of the microorganisms isolated from the test, the growth of this species (or these species) may be ascribed unequivocally to faults with respect to the material and/or the technique used in conducting the sterility test procedure.

The key word here is "unequivocally"—that is a huge burden of proof. Nucleic acid analyses may permit you to distinguish types among the same genus and species of organisms isolated from the manufacturing and testing suites (1,17). Anything less than nucleic acid analyses is unequivocal and cannot be used to distinguish origin differences between isolates of the same genus and species.

If an extensive investigation of the OOS looking for process, nonprocess, and laboratory errors concludes that the test was unequivocally contaminated in the laboratory and can be justifiably invalidated, the USP says that the new test should use the same sample size as the original test. However, USP does not allow for another invalidation should the repeat test be positive. A positive test on a postinvalidation sample "does not comply with the test for sterility."

Invalidating a test on a closed system where operator exposure to the test is minimized, or in an isolator, where operator intervention should be eliminated, is even more difficult than invalidating a test performed using an open system in a sterility test suite. In either of these two cases, the only rationale for invalidating a test is a documented failure in the system (e.g., loss of real pressure in the isolator or leak in the canister).

Media and Diluting Fluids

For the sterility test, the USP outlines specific procedures that a laboratory should use to demonstrate that each lot of medium, including the SCD, the FTM, and the diluting fluid used in the performance of the test meets the requirements for growth promotion and sterility (4). Validation in the form of the media sterility test and the growth promotion test will demonstrate the media's ability to support growth uniformly throughout the assigned expiration period. For media prepared in-house, this study must be performed for each type, presentation (e.g., plate size), and volume of medium (e.g., 10 mL of medium/tube, 100 mL of medium/tube). For media that is purchased, the assigned expiration dates of at least lots of media should be confirmed through the sterility and growth promotion tests as part of the initial vendor qualification studies. Sterility of the media along with its ability of to support growth is essential attributes of any microbiological medium.

Validation

The USP sterility test presumes that if contamination were to happen during manufacturing, and if a contaminated unit were to be sampled and tested, then the result of the test would be positive (i.e., growth of that organism would be observed during the 14-day incubation period).

The "Validation Test" described in USP< 71 >(4) requires that the analyst perform the sterility test in the manner described in the chapter (preferably MF), but instructs the analyst to add not more than 100 colony-forming units (CFU) of one of the indicator panel of organisms to the final rinse of the filtration process for the test article. Note that the organisms are added to the final rinse, not to the test article itself. The indicator panel represents a spectrum of organisms that might be found in a sterility test including organisms isolated from humans as well as from the environment and includes mold, yeast, Gram-positive and Gram-negative bacteria, aerobe, anaerobe, and facultative anaerobe. A parallel test without the test article, but using the same number of organisms is performed as a positive control. Test material + organism is incubated along with the positive control for not more than five days. After the incubation period, both the test and the positive control are visually observed, and the growth is compared. If the growth in the tube containing the test article is visually comparable to the positive control, the product possesses no antimicrobial activity relative to that organism, and the test may proceed. If growth observed in the presence of the product is visually less than the positive control, the product possesses some level of antimicrobial activity and the test method must be reevaluated to identify the cause of the interference. The method must be modified to eliminate or neutralize the antimicrobial activity. Interference may be eliminated by chemical inactivation (e.g., the use of penicillinase to inactivate penicillins and cephalosporins), the addition of a neutralizer such as Tween to the diluting fluid, and/or increasing the volumes and numbers of rinses to physically eliminate interfering substances that might remain on the membrane after filtration. For each sterile product, raw material, or intermediate under test, the validation test is repeated for each of the panel of indicator organisms. Many regulators expect that an environmental isolate or an organism isolated from a prior sterility OOS will be added to the panel of organisms used in the validation. Why use so many organisms for the validation? In addition to representing a number of different categories and sources of microorganisms, this variety of microorganisms represents a spectrum of sensitivities to common antimicrobial and sanitizing agents. For example, *Bacillus subtilis* spores could survive in the presence of residual ethanol, whereas *Pseudomonas aeruginosa* vegetative cells would be much more susceptible to the antimicrobial activity of ethanol. Organisms isolated from a cephalosporin-manufacturing environment is representative of organisms that are resistant to the effects of the antibiotic.

The USP sterility test does not require that a product be "spiked" with microorganisms and that those microorganisms be quantitatively or qualitatively recovered. Rather, the indicator organism, in low numbers, is added to the final rinse of the test. Therefore, the validation does not answer the question of recovering organisms that might contaminate the product during manufacture or filling, but rather it demonstrates that the test method, in particular, the inactivation or removal of any potentially inhibitory substances that might remain on the filter surface, will not present conditions where organisms are prevented from growing. This is perhaps a small distinction, but a very important one.

APPENDIX 2: THE STATISTICS OF ENDOTOXIN AND STERILITY TESTING

The sterility test and the bacterial endotoxin test, regardless of the result, provide extremely limited information on the presence or absence of contaminated units in a batch of a parenteral product. Sterility and absence of detectable endotoxin are assured, not through end-product testing, but through the careful execution of a series of well conceived and executed validation studies and value-added monitoring activities to demonstrate that the processes, including equipment, process stream, filling, environment, people, and appropriate test methods, are capable of consistently producing a product that is sterile and free of detectable endotoxin.

Case #1: Sterility Testing

If the result of a validated USP sterility test is negative, what can one say about the sterility of the batch? Let us assume we demonstrate via process simulation (media fill) studies that our inherent contamination rate is less than 1 in 1000 vials, and we take the prescribed 20 vials for our sterility test. A negative test result using a validated test method suggests that, to the limit of detection of the test, there were no contaminated vials in the 20 that we chose for our test sample. If our fill size were only 20 vials, we could reasonably conclude that our batch is sterile—however, we would have no product to sell. What does a negative sterility test mean when the batch size is much larger than the sample size—say 50,000 units?

As the total population of 50,000 units is much larger than our sample size, we need to approximate the probability of finding a contaminated vial using a statistical technique called binomial distribution. In order to use this technique, four requirements need to be met:

1. The experiment consists of n identical trials, where n is set in advance. For our sterility test, each sample vial is an identical trial, and the number of vials taken (20) is set by our SOP.
2. Each outcome can be categorized as either a success or a failure. For a sterility test, the contamination status of each vial is either sterile/negative (success) or contaminated/positive (failure).
3. The trials are independent—one trial does not affect the outcome of the other. In our test, each vial, although ultimately pooled for the purposes of the test, represents an independent trial, whereas the contamination status of the contents of one vial has no effect on the contamination status of another vial.
4. The probability of success must be constant from one test to the next. In our case, we have measured our inherent contamination rate as less than 1 in 1000 vials, so unless something in manufacturing changes, contamination rate should be consistent from process to process.

   We are interested in knowing the probability of getting one or more contaminated vials in our sample. In statistical terms, the probability of getting at least one contaminated vial is the same as one minus the probability of getting no positively contaminated vials.

$$P(X \geq 1) = 1 - P(X = 0)$$

To find the probability that no vial is contaminated, we use the formula:

$$P(x = 0) = (1 - \pi)^n$$

where π is the probability of a contaminated vial ($< 1:1000$) and n the number of units in our sample.

Calculating out, the probability of testing a contaminated vial is less than

$$1 - (1 - \pi^n) = 1 - (1 - 0.001)^{20} = 1 - (0.999)^{20} = 1 - 0.980189$$

or

$\leq 1.9\%$ chance of getting a positive test

In other words, given the conditions of the test described above, we have a 98% chance of passing the test!

This calculation tells us that there is less than a 2% chance of our finding a contaminated vial, given a batch size of 50,000, a sample size of 20, and an inherent contamination rate of less than 1 in 1000 units. Knowing that, one might ask the question, "How contaminated does the lot need to be in order for me to fail a sterility test assuming a batch size of 50,000 and a sample size of 20?" Table 5 provides the answer.

The statistics tells us that the contamination rate would have to be remarkably high result to in a 50% probability of failing the test. So, a positive on a validated USP sterility test would indicate either that the batch is highly contaminated (which should have an obvious root cause in a properly validated and controlled manufacturing process) or the test was inadvertently contaminated by the analyst. Which of the two scenarios will provide a root cause? Only an unbiased and scientific investigation will fulfill GMP requirements for an appropriate dispositions.

Case #2: Endotoxin Testing

The bacterial endotoxin test provides us with another mathematical challenge. The logic process for looking at the usefulness of an end-product endotoxin test is the same as for a sterility test, but some of the assumptions change.

1. Instead of 20 units/sample, the bacterial endotoxins test (BET) for a parenteral drug product usually requires only three samples, one each from the beginning, middle, and end of the run. So, our n is 3. Medical devices usually test 10 samples.
2. As with sterility, the outcome of the test is either a success or a failure. Success in the case of BET is endotoxin below the calculated or assigned endotoxin limit (pass). Failure is the detection of endotoxin in excess of the limit.
3. As with sterility, each unit represents an individual outcome, even though the contents of the vials might be pooled for our study.
4. We run into a problem when we try to assign a contamination rate for endotoxin, as there is no endotoxin analog to a process simulation/media fill. Unlike sterility testing, endotoxin testing is not visual in that we do not see a contamination event as turbidity in an incubated vial. To determine endotoxin contamination across the run, one would have to test every vial. Unlike sterility, endotoxin contamination is not an absolute. We cannot measure zero endotoxin, and in fact, we are allowed to have endotoxin in our product, but the measured level of endotoxin cannot exceed the calculated or assigned endotoxin limit.

If, for the sake of discussion that the endotoxin contamination rate approximates the microorganism contamination rate, then a 50,000 unit batch, assuming a 1 in 1000 contamination rate and a sample size of 30 calculates as follows:

$$P(x = 0) = (1 - \pi)^n$$

$$1 - (1 - \pi^n) = 1 - (1 - 0.001)^3 = 1 - (0.999)^3 = 1 - 0.997$$

or

$\leq 0.3\ \%$ chance of getting a positive test

In other words, given the conditions of the test described above (a sample size of 3, a batch size of 50,000, and a contamination rate of > 1 in 1000 units), we have a 99.7% chance of passing the test! Again, with such a low sample size relative to the batch size, finished product endotoxin testing tells us very little about the level of endotoxin in the batch of product. Monitoring the process using a risk analysis method such as HACCP (Chapter 8) will provide our company with much better endotoxin control than end product testing alone.

Index

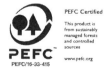
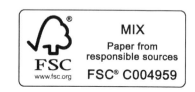
#0056 - 080515 - C0 - 229/152/14 [16] - CB